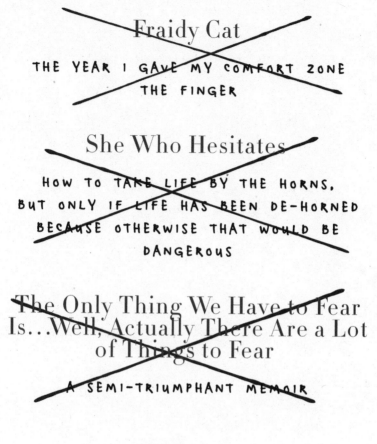

~~Fraidy Cat~~
~~THE YEAR I GAVE MY COMFORT ZONE THE FINGER~~

~~She Who Hesitates~~
~~HOW TO TAKE LIFE BY THE HORNS, BUT ONLY IF LIFE HAS BEEN DE-HORNED BECAUSE OTHERWISE THAT WOULD BE DANGEROUS~~

~~The Only Thing We Have to Fear Is…Well, Actually There Are a Lot of Things to Fear~~
~~A SEMI-TRIUMPHANT MEMOIR~~

Okay
Fine
Whatever

Okay
Fine
Whatever

THE YEAR I WENT FROM BEING AFRAID OF EVERYTHING TO ONLY BEING AFRAID OF MOST THINGS

Courtenay Hameister

Little, Brown and Company
New York   Boston   London

Little, Brown and Company
Hachette Book Group
1290 Avenue of the Americas, New York, NY 10104
littlebrown.com

First Edition: July 2018

Little, Brown and Company is a division of Hachette Book Group, Inc. The Little, Brown name and logo are trademarks of Hachette Book Group, Inc.

This work was made possible in part due to a grant from the Regional Arts and Culture Council, Portland, Oregon.

Author's note: Portions of essays in this book have appeared on *Live Wire!* radio and *Back Fence PDX*, in *Portland Monthly* magazine, *Oregon Humanities* magazine, and on *GoLocalPDX*.

The publisher is not responsible for websites (or their content) that are not owned by the publisher.

The Hachette Speakers Bureau provides a wide range of authors for speaking events. To find out more, go to hachettespeakersbureau.com or call (866) 376-6591.

ISBN 978-0-316-39570-0
LCCN 2017958219

10 9 8 7 6 5 4 3 2 1

LSC-C

Printed in the United States of America

Contents

CONTENTS

CONTENTS

For Mom and Scott—
Without you, I could never have accomplished
anything.

What I'm saying is, this is all your fault.

Okay
Fine
Whatever

Introduction:

Getting Plucky

Imagine you are eight years old.

You are at a community pool in Akron, Ohio, with your entire extended family—uncles, cousins, grandparents, and your older brother, whose opinion you hold in high regard because he can make realistic fart noises using his hand and armpit.

You have made the egregious mistake of climbing to the top of the high dive.

You are now standing at the edge of the diving board, looking down into the blue abyss miles below you.

Okay, like, sixteen feet below you.

It feels like you're about to jump out of a plane. Or off a bridge. Or into the ocean in *Jaws* after you've already seen that one unfortunate teenager get pulled under.

The fear feels insurmountable, but so does the ire of the five kids in line, including four on the ladder and one standing behind you at the other end of the board, glaring, his sun-kissed arms akimbo.

"Just *go!*" he whines.

His plea is one of dozens you've heard for the past ten minutes while staring into what, to everyone else, is a calm pool of welcoming blue water.

Finally, the tension becomes too much for your knocking knees, and you sit down at the end of the board, triggering frustrated sighs and expletives from every diver in line.

"You can do it, sweetie!" your mother yells, her hand poised in a blocking-the-sun salute. "It'll be over in a second. Just jump."

But you know something she doesn't.

It's too late.

You already know you can't do it, and now instead of working up the courage to jump, you're working up the courage to walk the gauntlet of searing side-eyes you'll endure on the Climb of Shame down to the scorching pavement.

This is where you learned it: You are not the leaping type.

This story is both a true account of the first time I disappointed the crap out of my older brother in public and an encapsulation of how I lived my life up until a couple years ago.

I was a toe-dipper. A cringer. A wait-and-see-er.

People wouldn't necessarily have known this, because through a heroic feat of white-knuckling, I managed to pass myself off as a regular, sometimes-relaxed, initiative-taking adult. And a high-functioning one, at that.

I had a cool job.

I hosted *Live Wire!*, a nationally syndicated public radio show wherein I interviewed fascinating people like Gus Van Sant, Tig Notaro, Mike Birbiglia, and Carrie Brownstein...and tried to keep from fear-puking while on air.

I was lucky, but I was also terrified. Every week I hosted the show, I looked like I was leaping, but I was still on that diving board and I hadn't moved an inch.

It wasn't just my job that caused me anxiety. Everything did.

Phone calls to strangers were miserable. Parties where I didn't know anyone were like the seventh circle of hell but with better snacks. And making an unprotected left turn triggered the same fight-or-flight response most people experience when running from a small- to medium-size bear.

You can imagine how all of this affected my romantic life. One side effect of my sometimes crippling anxiety: I didn't have an actual adult relationship until I was thirty-four. Not surprisingly, this turned out to create its own set of issues, which I'll get into later.

It wasn't until the poop hit the propellers at work in an epic, slow-motion, action-movie kind of way that I went to a counselor, who informed me that, in addition to the OCD I already knew about, I'd been struggling with generalized anxiety disorder for most of my life.

That meant that I had full-on OCD attacks pretty rarely, but my daily level of anxiety about things like work, relationships, finances (y'know, life?) was disproportionately high compared to that of other people.

And suddenly it all made sense: I wasn't a giant fucking wuss; I had a disease.

I had a disease that not only made me afraid to take chances but also turned me into an Eeyore in a world seemingly filled with Tiggers. Anxiety makes you think that nothing is going to go well, and eventually, that becomes a habit. Eventually, it's not just jumping out of a plane that might have disastrous consequences, it's also talking to the checker at the grocery store or just leaving the house.[1]

This book is about my attempt to climb out of the ruts in my neural pathways that said everything was going to suck. To rewire the negative connections that quashed any effort to change. To try things that scared me in order to teach my brain that everything was going to be okay.[2] It was my version of exposure therapy—to the entire world.

Spoiler alert: I didn't jump out of planes.

I did things that were frightening in more of a "Can embarrassment turn into a permanent condition?" way than an "I'm going to end up as a heap of bones at the bottom of the Grand Canyon" way. Things like, for instance, taking a fellatio class.

And speaking of oral sex, I didn't exempt dating from my project. I went on more dates in a year than I'd been on in my entire life, which, to be honest, wasn't that difficult to do.

I dubbed this my Okay Fine Whatever Project because *okay, fine,*

---

1   In my defense, thirteen people are killed every year by vending machines, so you never know what peril awaits you when you walk out that door.

2   Important disclaimer: This book was written prior to the 2016 election, when an undercurrent of ugliness in our culture was further revealed and encouraged. As a white woman in America, I realize it is great privilege that makes it possible for me to go out and pursue things that scare me, since just driving a car can be an act of courage for a person of color in this country. That being said, I believe that we all have self-doubt, anxiety, and fears that can be overcome, and I hope it's possible for everyone to find something of value in this book. If you don't, let me know on Twitter, which is now just the Digital Land of Angry People (note: I am one of them).

whatever are the words we anxious people utter when embarking on adventures that Tiggers might be excited about, like being dragged to a concert or on a trip or to our own Nobel Peace Prize award ceremony.

I wasn't kidding myself that I could magically turn into a brave person, but I hoped that, just maybe, I could become a not-constantly-scared person. A person who was less lonely, less gloomy, and who didn't feel like such a liar when she told herself that everything was going to be okay.

If you've ever struggled with anxiety, I offer this: Anxious people are braver than the un-anxious, because we do it anyway, every single day. We're faced with fear on a regular basis, and we push through it in order to simply live our lives. And that's something to be proud of.

Also, we're kind of lucky, we anxious few. Because when you're scared of everything, everything is an adventure.

So let the (sort of) adventure begin.[3]

---

3   A note about memoir and accuracy: Everything in this book happened, but the timing of some events has been shifted to improve narrative flow, and conversations presented are, of course, not word for word but how I remember them. Also, I swear like a sailor. Although my cousin was a sailor and he didn't seem to swear any more than anyone else in my family, so I guess I swear like a Hameister.

Stepping Down:

Wherein I Unknowingly Plant the Seeds for a Series of Tiny Adventures

Imagine[1] you're an accountant. (Or, if you're an accountant, imagine you're you.)

Now imagine[2] that numbers terrify you. Your pulse quickens and your throat closes up as you're buttoning your shirt for work in the morning. Brushing your teeth, you feel disconnected from reality as your mind races, picturing the thousands of numbers that await you on your computer screen. When you finally reach your desk and see all the spreadsheets laid out in front of you, you feel like someone has attached electrodes to your upper body and is slowly turning up the

---

1   I know I just told you to imagine you were eight years old, and now I'm taxing your imagination yet again. Just bear with me.

2   I promise this is the last time I'll ask you to work.

voltage. Your chest tightens and buzzes with energy, making it impossible to get a full breath.

If this happened to you every morning, you would never continue your accounting career. That would be madness.

Now imagine you're a performer prone to unpredictable bouts of stage fright.

Welcome to another day at work.

This was what show days felt like for me when I was hosting *Live Wire!*, a radio variety program that's recorded in front of a live audience in Portland, Oregon, and airs on about a hundred public radio stations nationally.

Every week, in the days leading up to the show, I felt the anxiety as more of a dull pain than a stabbing one. At each Monday writers' meeting, I would grimace as I felt the first stirrings in my chest of what I called my dread ball. The dread ball began its life the size of a pea, but by Wednesday, it was decidedly watermelonish, heavy and tight and filling my chest with a muffled smoldering that threatened to explode out of my lungs, which, it turns out, I needed in order to breathe. By show day—Saturday—my dread ball had turned into a giant, human-size hamster ball I'd walk around in, the rest of the world dulled by the view through the plastic.

I did lots of things on the show—read essays, performed in comedy sketches—and those things were sometimes great; fun, even. It was interviewing people in front of an audience that filled me with dread (balls). It's strange to meet someone for the first time in any situation—imagine doing it in front of four hundred people who paid good money to see a compelling conversation. And when every person you interview is a leader in his or her field: a Pulitzer

Prize–winning author, an Oscar-winning filmmaker, the creator of the wiki software, the stakes go even higher.

I never finished college, which is a bit of a sore spot for me, and it felt like once a week, I was sitting onstage holding up a huge arrow pointing to the giant hole where my education should've been. I was always worried I would seem like an idiot by comparison to my guests, which was in itself kind of idiotic, since I did tons of research on them prior to their arrival, and it's not like Bruce Campbell was going to come on the show and want to discuss *The Iliad*.[3]

I stuck it out, though, because I had lots of reasons to. I got to collaborate with insanely talented people who made me look way smarter than I was. I met extraordinary artists like David Rakoff, Cheryl Strayed, and Bob Odenkirk and got to ask them about their creative processes, which turned my job into a paid decade-long MFA program with a well-stocked craft-service table. And the best part: The show gave me essay-writing hard deadlines that would've resulted in public humiliation in front of an audience of four hundred to seven hundred if they were not met. The constant fear of this humiliation made me create more new work than most of the writers I knew.

So there were plenty of good reasons to stay as well as one not-so-good reason: the nagging, terrifying idea that this job was the most interesting thing about me.

I already knew I had trouble talking to strangers at parties, and my

---

3   Sure, some might see a correlation between the wrath of Achilles and the rage of Ash in the Evil Dead movies, but Achilles was largely driven by honor, whereas Ash was driven by the desire to blow the heads off zombies.

eHarmony profile had caused exactly three men in dad-jeans to beat a path to my digital door, so I didn't feel like I had a ton of personality traits to recommend me. This job caused me great angst, but it also gave me great anecdotes, and when someone asked me, "What do you do?," I could answer with a job title shared by only about three other people in the country.[4] That felt like a selling point for me.

Of course I realize I'm not a product, but when you're a single woman in your forties, it's difficult not to think of yourself as a brand. (*Tired of the everyday? Looking for something slightly divergent from the norm but not intimidatingly so? Try Courtenay! She's arty!*) And if I was a brand, my flagship product was the show.

Once I'd made the mistake of allowing my job to define me in that way, I could no longer consider quitting it without feeling like I would be quitting myself.

And then, on March 14, 2013, three days before our ninth-anniversary show, none of the identity stuff mattered because I was having a massive anxiety attack. Not a hit-and-run anxiety attack, but the kind that sits down and orders a double. The kind that wakes up with you and asks how you slept. The kind that laughs when you tell it that you have a show in three days and could it go bother Garrison Keillor, because he seems like a guy who could benefit from a little nervous energy. (And, apparently, a sexual-harassment workshop.)

---

4   Yes, I did fall into the somewhat large category of "radio host," but my category was whittled down to "host of a radio variety show" and then even further whittled down to "host of a radio variety show that records in front of a live audience." At the time, it was me, Garrison Keillor, and John Moe of *Wits*. Unless there was a large underground community of radio-variety-show hosts I was unaware of.

If you've never had an anxiety attack, it's a lot like that feeling you have when you almost get into a car accident or someone startles you. But what if that feeling just didn't go away? What if it hung around for hours or even days, like that one friend who won't leave your party and eats all the guacamole you were planning to binge on later?

In this case, the panic attack was triggered by an OCD episode, the second one of my life.

The first one happened a year after my father died.

My father was a good, kind, sometimes naive and awkward man who'd spent his entire adult life living with bipolar disorder. He'd gone to West Point and done two tours in Vietnam, and when he came back to the States at thirty-five, he decided that he wanted to be a doctor. So for most of my childhood, he was either out of the country, studying for med school, or working. Despite manic depression and dyslexia, he still managed to become a family practitioner and an army colonel, which was totally badass, but as you can imagine, some of the family stuff fell through the cracks.

My mother picked up more than her share of the slack, and she, my brother, and I became a sort of three-person unit that my father had trouble breaking into.

I was a particularly sensitive and neurotic child (read: "giant pain in the ass"), so I took his absences personally. When I was in college, he reached out to me and my brother, trying to create a relationship. My brother reached back. I didn't.

When I was twenty-seven, my father pulled into a Holiday Inn parking lot and took a pill that he knew would stop his heart. He died within minutes.

The guilt I felt was immediate and crushing.

I left school in Texas and went to live with my mother in the southern mountains of Colorado.

I'd lived there about a year when the OCD hit. I was spending the weekend in a tree house built by some friends of my mother's that sat at the top of a butte with 360-degree views of the San Juan Mountains. It was a completely inappropriate place to fall apart.

Some people's OCD manifests as compulsive rituals, like handwashing to get rid of germs or repeatedly driving around the block to make sure you didn't hit anyone your last time around. These activities are all triggered by intrusive thoughts—irrational thoughts you don't want and can't control that shove their way into your psyche like a lesser Kardashian at a *Vanity Fair* Oscar party.

My version of OCD was just the intrusive thoughts without the compulsions. There are different versions of intrusive-thought OCD, and mine was harm-focused (HOCD), the sort wherein your mind convinces you that you've done something awful, like stabbed or killed someone, but you can't for the life of you come up with what you did.

During that first episode after my father died, I imagined that I'd harmed some kids I used to babysit. While I sat in the upstairs loft of the tree house looking out on perhaps the most glorious sunset of my life, I meticulously combed through every memory I had of babysitting them, but nothing ever surfaced. This, it turns out, is a classic symptom of HOCD.

The terrible thing about HOCD's intrusive thoughts is that your mind and body respond as if you've done the terrible thing you're imagining. The crime may be fictional, but the guilt, the fear, and the shame are all too real. And so is the massive, crippling anxiety.

Imagine the worst thing you could ever do. Now imagine you think you actually did it.

That.

It turns out these OCD episodes tend to happen to me in times of great stress or when I urgently need to make a huge change in my life and am avoiding doing so.

In this case, I'd lived with my mother for a year in this tiny little town in the mountains and it was time to go, but fear and inertia wouldn't allow me to. Enter a crippling OCD episode.

Now, back to my second OCD episode, in 2013. This time, three days before the *Live Wire!* ninth-anniversary show, I began to worry I would harm my roommate, Shelly.

Shelly is perhaps the best person I know. She's a small, supersonic rocket of a woman—a pixie-like ball of energy, joy, and generosity who works as a web developer by day and an assemblage artist by night.

Thinking you might harm her is like thinking you might harm a baby kangaroo or that elf from *Rudolph* who just wanted to be a dentist.

These episodes are crippling because it's difficult to function when you believe you're the worst person in the world. When you wake up in the morning, you've forgotten that you are, but your OCD reminds you and the pattern starts again—obsess, reassure yourself, breathe deeply and feel almost normal, then remember that there are knives in the kitchen that you have access to.

My version of OCD has never caused me to imagine anything specific; it only gives me the idea that something might have happened or might happen. It's extraordinary that something so vague could be so terrifying, but the mind is magical in super-fucked-up ways.

So, back to my celebratory ninth-anniversary anxiety attack. It was the night before the show, and the panic was still living in every inch of my skin and bones. It was inside of me and I was inside of it simultaneously, and neither of us was going anywhere anytime soon.

And while my biggest concern was how to quell this panic, my second-biggest concern was how to function onstage with a mind this otherwise occupied.

That night, I went to my brother's house. With a psychology degree and decades as a bartender, Scott knows how to listen and calm people down regardless of the state they're in—an ability that is greatly appreciated by all the "creative types" who know and love him. He has this trick when you're arguing with him in which he repeats what you just said in an even, quiet voice that makes you realize that you might be overreacting or being hypersensitive or slightly on the batshit-crazy side. It's very effective and often quite humbling.[5]

I explained what was happening and he calmly told me I didn't have any choice but to cancel the show. I told him I couldn't cancel because too many people were counting on me.

Scott has always been the one person in my life willing to be brutally honest with me.

He gave me a little smile that said *While it's adorable how important you think you are, the earth will actually keep spinning if you cancel,* and he handed me the phone.

---

5   He once asked me to sneak a bag of popcorn into the dollar movies, and we argued about it quite heatedly. I yelled at him that I didn't want to get caught. "How would you get caught?" he asked. I told him that they would smell the popcorn in my backpack. He looked at me and slowly repeated what I'd said. "They're going to...smell the popcorn...in your bag...at the *movie theater.*" See? Humbling.

I called the producer and, for the first time in nine years, told her I couldn't perform the next night. I also offered her a solution: One of the guests we were planning to have on, Luke Burbank, an incredibly quick-witted, charming, natural showman who hosted his own popular podcast, could fill in. We'd actually booked him to see if he'd be a good replacement for me if I ever got sick, so it made perfect sense to try him out, since I was, if you consulted the *Diagnostic and Statistical Manual of Mental Disorders,* currently very sick.

The next night, the worst and the best thing happened: The show was utterly, completely fine without me. That sucked. And it was wonderful. But it also sucked.

Luke glided through the show as if he'd been hosting it all along, and I could suddenly breathe.

For a couple agonizing weeks, my friends, family, and colleagues watched me struggle to make the decision they'd seen coming for years. In the end, I stepped down as host and remained head writer and co-producer. I felt my body change the moment I decided. My shoulders relaxed, my chest opened up, and my stomach became virtually knot- and butterfly-free.

The only time the decision truly leveled me was after the first show I spent at the producers' table, a month after I'd stepped down.

The night had gone quite smoothly—in fact, it was amazing to watch a show without the dread ball ruining it for once. I was entertained, I did my job well, and I was frankly quite proud of myself for handling what could've been an awkward situation with aplomb.

Afterward, we all went to the bar across the street from the theater as we always did. The crowd there was usually a mix of show guests, staff, and audience members. I sat down at the bar and ordered a drink.

I turned around to see who else was there and spotted Luke sitting at a banquette in the corner, talking to the film director who had been a guest. There were a few people surrounding them, listening. Luke was holding court.

I remembered how I'd felt after every one of the two hundred shows I'd hosted: A tidal wave of relief with a few droplets of pride in it would wash over me as soon as I heard the final theme music and the audience applause died down. Then I'd walk out to the beaming faces of friends who had come to see the show, and strangers would approach me to thank me for a great night, or tell me their favorite parts, or say they knew people from my past, like a guy I'd worked in advertising with or punched at a party in the late nineties.[6]

A lot of people don't get to enjoy post-spotlight moments like this, and yet I don't think I handled them well; I deflected all compliments with ninja reflexes. I felt strange about getting positive feedback because I generally wasn't responsible for the best moments of the night—or any of the moments, for that matter. The show was put together by a crew of producers and writers and musicians and staff, and I was just another member of that troupe. But I got to stand in the spotlight for three hours and then step out of it and have everyone attribute the whole production to me, for good or for bad.

When I saw Luke holding court, I realized that I was witnessing what I had really lost: All that gratitude, all that admiration—all those people believing that I had my shit together and that I was worthy of three

---

6   I never punched anyone in the nineties (or ever). That just sounds more interesting than what I actually did in the nineties, which was watch a lot of *Friends* and not get laid.

hours of their time. I had relied on that gratitude and admiration, though I had never figured out how to accept it gracefully. And now I'd lost that four-hundred-person affirmation that, unbeknownst to me, I'd been using to counteract all the dickish things I said to myself every day.

I realized all of this in one terrible moment at the bar, and Jim, a friend and one of the show's producers, saw it happen.

"You okay?" he asked.

"Yep," I said, and I bolted to the bathroom, managing to lock the door behind me before the tears fell.

I sat on the toilet and sobbed as the weight of the decision crashed down on me.

I rocked back and forth and read the graffiti on the bathroom wall to try to distract myself.

Joshua West is a selfish prick.

You are worthy.

I ate too much cheese.

I laughed a little and pulled myself together, but then my brain refocused on the trigger image (some Seattle rando[7] basking in a glow that used to belong to me), as it was wont to do.

And more crying.

I was fine after about seven minutes, but now the problem was my face.

It looked like a map of Russia and the former Yugoslavia with a pair of frog eyes to the north and a clown nose where Bulgaria should be.

The only way I could get out of there without Luke seeing me was

---

7   He is not a Seattle rando. He is a very nice man. I was upset.

to make a run for it. I speed-walked to the bar to grab my purse, keeping my back to him. That meant facing two of the show's producers, but that was fine because I'd known them for a decade and they were already aware that I was a colossal crybaby.

Jim followed me outside.

"Hey," he said. "They still love you. They all still love you."

I felt so pathetic for being a person who needed to hear something like that.

"No," I said. "They don't. They don't even see me anymore."

Those faceless crowds of people didn't know me and I didn't know them, but obviously they'd meant more to me than I'd been willing to admit to myself.

To be clear, I've never missed the actual job, but I will always miss everything and everyone the job brought me.

And it made me wonder: Why couldn't I push through the anxiety and just enjoy the job?

I asked that question of William Todd Schultz, a friend who's a professor of psychology and the author of *Torment Saint: The Life of Elliott Smith*. He attributed it to my personality type—high in neuroticism and low in extroversion.[8] Shocker: Those two things don't go well with performing. (*Welcome to the show, everyone! Also, fuck you, I'm leaving, this is horrible.*)

Extroverts thrive on external stimulation (like hundreds of clapping people), while introverts get their energy from time spent alone

---

8   I took a test online that rates you on the Big Five personality traits, and he was right on both counts. I recommend you take it too! It's illuminating. And sometimes depressing. But it might not be depressing for you. You're probably perfect! Seriously, you seem nice.

and are far more sensitive to stimuli (like hundreds of clapping people). Some level of extroversion is obviously important for a performer. And, according to Schultz, being high in neuroticism is particularly problematic for entertainers, as it leads to more pronounced anticipatory dread, which, as we know, was kind of my jam.

I asked Luke, the guy who took my place as host, what made it worthwhile for him to get up onstage, as he always looked completely at ease—sometimes more than when he wasn't onstage. "It's been said to me by people I'm married to that I'm much better at relating to large groups," he quipped. "And there's a reason for that. Your good interactions with a single person—imagine sort of mainlining the best uncut freaking adrenochrome of that. It's euphoric."

I also talked to Ophira Eisenberg, the host of NPR's *Ask Me Another* and a longtime stand-up comic, and she put it this way: "When I'm not onstage for a while, I get a little grumpy," she said. "I can feel that my sense of myself is affected by the audience's reaction to me. And that's a little fucked up, but if it's your job to be propelled forward by positive reactions, doesn't it naturally become part of who you are? So there's a portion of my love for myself that's decided by a bunch of drunk people in a basement, and I just have to live with that."

I can relate to both of them. Just because I am, as Todd put it, "temperamentally ill-equipped to be onstage" that doesn't mean I don't crave connection. I recently saw a picture of myself walking offstage after reading an essay on *Live Wire!*, and I was shocked. The expression on my face looked like pure, unadulterated joy, but that's not what I remember when thinking of a show. The part I remember most is the week of trepidation I felt before each show for the very reason Eisenberg mentions: I believed that my success, failure, or worth as a person was going to be decided by four hundred people I didn't know. Sure, I might have a successful show, but successful enough to make up for the seventy-eight hours I spent worrying? It's like cooking Thanksgiving dinner—if you were to see the actual work-to-enjoyment ratio of that meal, you would never do it again. But almost none of us look at it that way; it's a matter of perspective.

And Eisenberg's and Burbank's perspectives are both unquestionably positive. In fact, almost pathologically so. When Ophira told her first stand-up joke ever, one person laughed. One. She described it as the biggest rush of her life. I asked her why she was so thrilled at what sounded to me like a sink-into-the-floor moment.

"The laugh was from someone I didn't know, so I saw that as success," she said. "Some people have 'laugh ears,' where they hear laughs that aren't there. Other people don't hear laughs that *are* there and come off the stage destroyed."

I was definitely in the latter group.

Unlike Burbank. "In stand-up, you only remember the people who laughed," he said. "I would record a set I thought was killing and replay it to hear three people laughing. It's a survival technique the spirit employs." You don't do the math, he said, otherwise you realize you're having a .05 percent success rate.

As for me, I could never *not* do the math. I am what psychologist Nancy Cantor referred to as a defensive pessimist: a person who doesn't necessarily expect the worst to happen but who prepares for it just in case. (*Sure, we probably won't get in a debilitating or disfigur-*

ing accident on the way to the 7-Eleven, but just in case we do, I'm going to press 9 and 1 on my phone so that once we crash, all I'll need to do is dial one number.) The problem is, defensive pessimism won't get you through weekly three-hour performances. You need to be able to push through the fear and the nerves and the YouTube comments over and over and over. You need what Luke and Ophira have in spades: a powerful, down-to-your-bones belief that in the end, everything is going to be okay.

I didn't have that feeling. I didn't think that I'd ever had it.

So when, during that epic anxiety attack, my body and mind seemed to be turning on me, in actuality they were trying to save me. If I'd continued hosting the show, I probably would've eventually had a heart attack. Maybe some things are worth dying for, but applause isn't one of them.

In the months that followed, as I eased into my new role at work, I noticed myself becoming increasingly unsettled. Not hosting the show created a huge mental chasm where worry used to live, and now I needed to fill it.

At the same time, I was frustrated by the fact that my anxiety had finally taken something huge from me. I'd always lied to myself, told myself it was manageable. Sure it was—in the same way that a stubborn cowlick or a white tiger is manageable. Which is to say, manageable until it ruins your sixth-grade class picture or rips half your neck out.

And this job wasn't the only thing anxiety had taken from me. It also took away my optimism. Living with a constant, low-buzzing anxiousness can rob you of your ability to imagine good things happening, or even recognize them when they do. You're always waiting for the other Croc to drop. (Things are dark in your imagination. Everyone wears Crocs.)

I started thinking about ways to get beyond my anxiety that didn't involve psychopharmaceuticals or hours of talk therapy, ways I might slowly teach my brain that fight-or-flight wasn't the correct response to every single situation. Could I reintroduce myself to the world? Show myself, like one shows a baby, which things were there for fun and edification, which were there to attack me with a knife, and how not to get the two confused?

Was it possible to relearn optimism?

That's when the Okay Fine Whatever Project was born.

I realized that if left to my own devices, I would spend most of my time either huddled in my house binge-watching Netflix or out with friends ordering the same drinks and hummus plates we always ordered even though what we really wanted was cheesy tots but since shame-eating wasn't a group activity, fuck it, we got hummus. I needed some external force acting on me to get me to escape my hummus prison.

I thought if I could create a situation in which I had to try new things for work, I might actually become braver. I might be able to get outside my hair-trigger brain and see things it hadn't allowed me to see before. I might even eventually become a badass.

I wrote to a friend who was an editor at a local website and proposed an idea for a column: I would do things that scared me and then write about them.

I would call my column the Reluctant Adventurer.

These were baby steps. I was not riding over Niagara Falls in a barrel. Not dropping everything and hiking the Pacific Crest Trail by myself.

Not even hiking Mill Ends Park by myself.[9] My goal was simply to try some things I wouldn't normally try. To do some things that caused me mental discomfort when I imagined them. In doing the show, I'd over-shot my mind's acceptable level of adventure by a bit. I just needed to scale it down.

I asked my editors to keep an eye out for comfort-zone-expanding experiences. I made my own list of activities in Portland that might fit the bill: Naked ecstatic dance (I hated my body). Sensory-deprivation tanks (I'm claustrophobic and afraid of the dark). A professional cuddler (oh my God, where to start?). Activities that wouldn't trigger a full-on anxiety attack but would make the pessimist in me throw a mini-tantrum before finally saying, *Okay! Fine. Whatever. I'll do it.*

That's how my Year of Living (Relatively) Dangerously[10] began.

---

9   Mill Ends Park is located in the middle of the median strip of Naito Parkway, a busy downtown thoroughfare in Portland, Oregon. At two feet across and a to-tal of 452 square inches, it's the world's smallest park. I still haven't hiked it.

10 In truth, it was more like a year and five months, but *A Year and a Half* doesn't look great on a book cover. People like nice, clean quantities of time. A day. A month. A millennium. Who wants to ride in the *Millennium-Ish Falcon?* No one.

The Sensory-Deprivation Tank:

In Which I Spend a Terrifying Ninety Minutes in a Bath of Warm Water

How would you like to spend ninety minutes in a tiny, pitch-black pod floating in warm water?

"Oh, that sounds wonderful," some of you might say, or "Oooh! So relaxing! I'd love to have some time away from my screaming kids!"

Perhaps you're people who enjoy spending time with yourselves. Personally, I'd had it up to here with my shit, and the thought of spending ninety minutes alone with me sounded like a not-so-fresh hell.

A few years ago, Sherry Turkle, an MIT professor who studies our relationship to technology, did a TED talk that rang a little too true for me. In it, she said that we, as a culture, have turned being alone into "a problem that needs to be solved." Whenever we're alone for two seconds, we pick up our phones so we don't have to hang out with our thoughts. In her book *Alone Together* she wrote that "we fill our days with ongoing connection, denying ourselves time to think and dream." I agree that what we're missing out on is reflection—actually considering our lives and the people in them. How we want to spend our time. Pursuing new ideas. Imagining a better, Angry Bird–less future.

And I do miss thinking, sure, but the reason I've given it up is that, for me, solitude is a chance for my brain to really immerse itself in regret.

Given the opportunity, I love to take time to regret how long it took me to become a "serious writer." I regret allowing myself to get heavy in college. I regret being financially irresponsible and unable to buy a house before Portland's housing boom began, back when I could've gotten a $500,000 house for $150,000. I regret not flossing. I regret the tax debt I incurred when I was freelancing. I regret the years I lost to heartbreak. I regret the bilevel haircut I got when I was a sophomore in high school.

I usually finish it all off by imagining what it'll be like to die homeless and alone because of my mental illness and all the financial and personal mistakes I've made.

That sort of thing.

That's why I take my phone to bed with me.

You cannot take your phone with you into the sensory-deprivation tank, which was a problem. Also, I am claustrophobic. I don't know why. I do remember that when I was nine, my brother pinned me down by sitting on my chest and dangled a string of spit from his mouth over my face and then sucked it back in at the last second. (For those of you who don't have older brothers, this is a thing they do. There should be a name for it—the Retractable Loogie? The Saliva

Psych-Out? Literal Torture That Should Be Covered by the Geneva Conventions but Isn't Because Families Aren't Countries?) I remember feeling trapped and getting panicked back then, but who wouldn't get panicked in that situation?

The only sensory-deprivation tanks I'd ever seen were the slightly-larger-than-human-size ones in the 1980 movie *Altered States,* and those looked like my worst trapped-in-an-abandoned-freezer nightmare. So the claustrophobia seemed like a problem.

And one last issue—I've been overweight most of my life. Which brings us back to regret and why it's difficult to be naked with myself for long periods. (If it weren't for the fact that I don't own a pair of cutoffs, I'd join Tobias Fünke in the Never Nudes.)

But even with all these reasons *not* to sign up, and despite my trepidation, I was a little intrigued by the idea when a friend who knew I was looking for activities outside my comfort zone suggested I try a sensory-deprivation tank. I did not run screaming but girded my loins. This seemed perfect for early in the Okay Fine Whatever Project. I'd heard it was relaxing and that there were a number of benefits, particularly for "creative people."[1]

Supposedly, when you cut out all sensory input, you can deactivate the lizard part of your brain,[2] the part that's always on the alert for a

---

1   I put that in quotes because actually labeling myself a creative person feels a little douche-y. Most people are creative as hell whether they know it or not; think of the acting job you did the last time you called in sick or faked an orgasm. I've opened office refrigerators and found warning Post-its on tuna-salad sandwiches that were as chilling as a Stephen King novel. Those were some creative sandwich-protectors.

2   Also known as the limbic system, which *Psychology Today* claims handles the six Fs: fight, flight, feeding, fear, freezing-up, and fornication.

dude with a knife or a co-worker with a metaphorical knife or a lump somewhere a lump shouldn't be. Once that "Holy crap, I'm gonna die" part of your brain quiets down, the rest of it is free to imagine great things. Or, in my case, to wonder why Pharrell Williams thinks a room without a roof is happy. (There are only three essential components to a room—walls, floor, roof—and it's missing a really important one. If that room is happy, that room is kidding itself.)

I chose to go to a place in Portland on Hawthorne Boulevard, a former hippie enclave. It was called Float On, and it billed itself as "America's Largest Float Tank Center." (There were six tanks to choose from, so apparently the bar isn't that high, America.)

I walked into a warm, inviting, deep blue waiting room with plush couches and tea on offer to calm me down before I went in and calmed down. The vibe was a lot like that of an acupuncture studio or a spa. It was quiet. Too quiet.

In terms of float-tank size, I was in sort of a Goldilocks situation, if Goldilocks were claustrophobic. There was the Oasis Tank, which looked like a combination of a space pod and a giant George Foreman Grill. I imagined if I got into one of those, I'd immediately have an anxiety attack. Which felt like the opposite of the point, so I skipped that one.

The next size up was the Float Pool, which allowed for a more open experience, if by *open experience,* one meant "as if you'd built a nice, clean mini-pool in the crawl space in your basement." That did not feel relaxing to me either.

The last size, the one I chose, was called the Ocean Float. It was about five feet by seven feet and allowed a person to stand when entering and exiting, so it was great for claustrophobics like myself or for anyone who's ever been locked in a car trunk and so might be a little jumpy. (Pro tip: If you're going to be abducted and thrown into a trunk, choose an abductor whose car was built in 2002 or after—all of these cars have lighted interior trunk releases. If your abductor's car is pre-2002, use your extra smartphone, which you've placed in a ziplock and shoved into an orifice just in case, to Google *How can I escape from the trunk of a car?* There's a wikiHow on it. For reals.)

Back to my float room: I was surprised at how clean and inviting it was. I walked into a ten-by-five anteroom with an open shower on one side and a set of wooden shelves with a lamp and all the supplies I'd need on the other. Supplies included earplugs to keep the salt water from getting into my ears, petroleum jelly to cover any recent cuts, and a white robe hanging on the back of the door, because you're supposed to float totally nude. (Side note for those who think floating in a pool other people have been in is gross: This particular location filters the water three times after each person and uses UV light to sanitize it.)

On the right side of the room was the space-age-looking pod door to the tank. It was about four feet tall and sat about two feet up from the floor. As soon as I opened it, the purple-blue glow of the UV light poured out. I peeked my head in to see a deep blue pool, stone-tile walls, and a blue ceiling covered in tiny lights that looked like stars. This was comforting for me, as I'm still a little afraid of the dark. Especially when I'm in pitch-black pools of water that could suddenly fill with miniature eels that swim into your ear canals and eat your brain.

I took off the robe at the very last possible second, crouched down, and stepped into the tank, the bottom of which was smooth, like a giant bathtub.

Marco at the front desk had told me that once you pull the door to your tank closed, get in, and turn the lights out, you're in complete blackness.

Well, you are if you remembered to turn the light in the shower room off like Marco reminded you to. If you forgot that, you'll step into the tank, lie down, turn out the tank lights, notice that light is seeping in from outside, say, "Fucking goddamn it," get up, step out of the pod door sopping wet and, risking electrocution, flick the lamp switch, get back in, and lie down again, and *then* you are floating in complete blackness. And steeped in slight annoyance, now tinged with anxiety because of the pitch-blackness.

In the same way I can't really explain my claustrophobia, I've never been able to explain my discomfort with pitch-blackness. Had there been another person in the room with me, I would've felt fine, like there was someone in there to protect me from whatever my lizard brain imagined was in the blackness. But alone in the darkness? That always made me feel like I was in a room that I knew had a spider in it somewhere but I couldn't see it.

It's an odd sensation when your heart starts to move up toward your throat even though you're doing something that's specifically designed to calm it down. And you can't just tell your body it's going in the wrong direction and should pull a U-ie.

I lay there in the (calming?) blackness and I breathed deep into my belly until my heart was back where it belonged. I know it drives people crazy when they're upset and someone tells them to breathe; it drives me crazy too. But at this point, we all need to suck it up and admit that the whole inhale-exhale thing is not woo-woo; it's science. Deep breathing triggers the parasympathetic nervous system, which tells your fight-or-flight response that everything's okay. It also oxygenates the blood and causes the brain to release endorphins, those same feel-good hormones that convinced you that you were in love with that guy who played opposite you in *South Pacific* in high school.

After about ten minutes of deep breaths 'n' calming thoughts, I felt like I was finally starting from where a "normal" person might start. Just eighty minutes to go.

I checked in with my body.

The pools are filled with water heated to 93.5 degrees, which is skin-receptor neutral, making it difficult to feel where your body ends and the water begins. If this freaks you out, you can reach over with one hand and touch your other hand to make sure it's still attached. I didn't need to do this because I'm not afraid of spontaneously losing a limb. Just the eel thing.

The water is mixed with eight hundred and fifty pounds of Epsom salt, which causes you to float in a decidedly "Sandra Bullock in *Gravity* but without the terror of impending death" kinda way. As someone who has struggled with weight issues her whole life, I cannot stress enough the relief that weightlessness brings. It's a version of what you get in a pool, but it's effortless (you can float a bit in a normal pool too, but eventually, unless you're on a raft, you're going to have to tread water). You just lie there and the water holds you up. And you can't look down and see what's sticking out of the water and kick yourself for that last burrito.

I could feel where the water ended on the spots where my body was exposed to air (the air was supposed to be the same temperature as the water but felt slightly cooler to me), but I couldn't see these areas, which I was grateful for.

And suddenly I remembered that I used to love swimming more than just about anything—the freedom from carrying all that excess weight, the ability to move in any direction, flowing with the water. Most people are graceful in a pool, as long as they know how to swim. (Drowning people are not very graceful. No offense if you're currently drowning.)

I loved swimming, that is, until one day in high school when French Club spent the day at a pool in Salinas, California. (Yes, I was in French Club. We were like the cool kids if the cool kids had been very uncool and spoke broken French.)

We were all taking turns doing silly dives, and as I stood on the diving board, bending my knees in preparation for a jump, Tom Fletcher, who would've been crowned high-school Snark King if that'd been a thing, began singing Thomas Dolby's 1980s techno-nerd anthem "She Blinded Me with Science" but changed the line "It's poetry in motion" to "She's cellulite in motion." (Nice meter match, dick.)

Cool song. Miserable memory.

I vaguely recall I'd felt pretty that afternoon until then.

Now what I mostly remember is the humiliation right before I hit the water. And then wanting to stay under until everyone went home. I did stay under for as long as I could, but I finally had to accept that this wasn't really a feasible solution to the problem.

Once I came up, I could feel the heat of shame on my face while my body remained cool and, more important, hidden under the water.

I asked my best friend, Jennifer, to bring my towel to the ladder at the deep end.

"Whatever, Your Highness," Jennifer said as she handed it over.

I flashed back to another diving-board moment seven years earlier when we were visiting family in Florida and my cousin Sarah yelled, "Look out! The elephant's about to jump in the pool!" That one stung too, despite what a lame dig it was. An elephant jumping in a pool? Elephants don't even spend that much time near water. What about "Look out! The whale's about to breach!" or "Oh no! They're lowering the *Titanic!*" She had so many water-related-insult options.

But even dumb insults have power. I rushed past our parents, who were drinking daiquiris in the kitchen, and spent a wet, cold hour crying behind a chair in her family's dark, air-conditioned living room. I kept replaying the moment in my head—mostly the part where my brother hadn't stood up for me.

I remember wanting so much to make Sarah feel as terrible as she'd made me feel. At the time, I was nine, so my go-to burn was *not* thanking a person in my future Oscar speech: *And I definitely don't want to thank my cousin Sarah...*

Cut to a few decades later, and through the magic of family reunions and a horrible thing called Facebook, I would come to learn that both my cousin and Tom Fletcher had gained weight. It was exactly what nine- and sixteen-year-old me would've wanted, but I didn't feel better. I just felt bad for all of us.

I want so much to be one of those women who feel great about their bodies, no matter their size. These women are self-actualized. They're badasses. They're miracles, in fact. To be able to flout a lifetime of messages that your thighs are an abomination unto God, that your dimpled cheeks are adorable but your dimpled ass is gag-inducing, and that your pretty face is wasted on your big body is, to me, miraculous.

I was always a hypersensitive kid, which I now attribute to my GAD (generalized anxiety disorder). Without GAD or another disorder working its magic, if someone says something horrible to you, you might find it easy to laugh it off. But the anxious person hears a dig and the brain goes immediately to *She's right. Of course she's right. How can I fix this? If I don't fix this, no one will ever love me.*

So it made perfect sense to me that in a spacious, belonging-to-everybody world, the fact that I took up too much space was an affront to everyone. And it also made sense that my punishment for this affront was to be invisible when I wanted to be seen and all too visible when I didn't. ("You're fat, but I'll fuck you!" a man once yelled at me in the middle of a crosswalk on West Fourth Street in New York. It was the most concise insult/threat-disguised-as-a-compliment I'd ever heard.)

At various times in my adult life, I've been a size 12, a 24, a 14, and an 18. I've run the size gamut and I've lost weight healthfully and horribly.

Ever hear someone say "I wish I were as fat as I was the first time I thought I was fat"? That sentence evokes every photo ever taken of me that I hated at the time but look back on with yearning, envying the person I was.

Thankfully, I eventually lost my train of body-shaming thought in the tank, but not before I noted that diving boards were just a horrible milieu for me. I obviously needed to stay away from them.

I'd be amazed if someone were able *not* to think about her body in the tank, because floating while sensorially deprived is the strangest mix of being disconnected from your body, in that you don't register gravity or see its shape, and being more connected to it than you've ever been.

More connected, because when everything else goes away, all that's left is what you feel, inside and outside your skin. All you can hear is your own breath—and not the almost-silent version you get while walking around day to day. It's the super-fresh amplified dance mix you get when your head is underwater, like you're listening to yourself huffing into a microphone for ninety minutes. And in that fraction of a second when your breath runs out, you hear your heart.

It was a soul-soothing soundtrack.

I moved my leg to feel the soft whoosh of the salt water as it passed over my skin. I adjusted my neck and heard every tiny crack as my spine shifted and my body got acclimated to weightlessness. My arms bobbed at my sides, and I did my best to remain motionless so I could feel what it was like to lose touch with the edges of my body. What would it be like not to live in a body? To just float through the world without a sense of where I began and ended? What would I have to obsess about every day? What would I count instead of calories?

I pulled my right arm out of the water and placed it on my stomach, feeling the cooler air as my belly rose and fell. After a few minutes, I could feel my skin tighten as the salt dried. I put my arm back in the water and mentally visited every body part, telling it to relax. I generally walked around in a state of constant tightness, like every muscle was scowling, flinching, waiting for a blow that never came. So each body part, after being visited and asked to calm down, noticeably relaxed toward the floor of the tank.

Once my body was relaxed, I had to deal with my brain.

It was still running at its normal pace, and it was all over the place. Some deep thoughts, some as shallow as the Epsom-salt-infused water I was floating in:

- Why do we have ear wax?
- What're those weird colored lights you see when your eyes are closed?[3]
- I wonder if people masturbate in these things. Should I masturbate? Would it make the experience better? Am I even in the mood? I don't think I am. Am I rejecting my own advances right now?
- What does salt water do to a vagina? Will mine look younger after this?
- When does your brain ever rest? Even when you're asleep, it's busy making dreams. That seems like a bummer of a job.
- My job's kind of a bummer right now. Should I have just left when I stepped down as host? What do I bring to the show anymore?
- What will I have to be proud of if I leave?
- Am I even proud of my work anymore?
- If I don't have kids, what am I leaving the world?
- I need to get grape tomatoes if I'm gonna make that salad for Marie's dinner.
- Why do we have organs in our body that can just be taken out without any consequences?

At one point, I think about thirty minutes in, my brain started quieting down, largely because the only input it was getting was the sound of my own heart and breathing. It makes sense that hearing

---

3   Those are phosphenes, which are colored patterns or stars created by the retina, which still produces electrical charges even when it's supposed to be resting (when you're in complete darkness). I guess our retinas are easily bored.

and feeling the rhythm that's been with me my whole life had a calming effect.

About an hour in, my brain shut up and I went into a state of just... quiet.

This was new.

It was, shockingly, kind of lovely and not at all what I'd imagined when I thought about what spending ninety minutes with myself would be like.

Many people say that they have creative epiphanies in the tanks, or they hallucinate (those might be phosphenes), or they rise to a new level of consciousness. I didn't have an epiphany, but I did feel more grounded when I walked out of that tank.

I'm not sure why I didn't epiphanize. It could be that when someone starts off as a nervous wreck, it's hard to get to a state of euphoria in ninety minutes. I might need longer to get there than your average person.

More than anything else, though, floating disconnected me from my screwed-up idea of my body and connected me to my actual body, which I generally avoid thinking about or touching or looking at in a mirror, mostly because I've spent my life treating it like I have a spare one somewhere.

I dream of being at peace with my weight every single day, so it's not surprising that the first time I'd found peace in a long time was while I was weightless.

The question was, how could I get to that serene place on dry land? Maybe my Okay Fine Whatever Project could help me get there. Taking a step outside my comfort zone hadn't hurt me so far, but I was just beginning. The mental jury was still out.

Recently, my friend Jennifer from high school posted an old picture of me on Facebook. It was taken on that humiliating day with French Club. I was sitting in a lounge chair in my new white bathing suit that had little ruffles at the hips, raising my arm to block my freckled face from the sun, and smiling broadly at the camera.

When I saw the picture, I wished so much that I could go back in time and talk to my sixteen-year-old self and say, "Hey, I just came back to let you know that in the future, a thing called Facebook will be invented and it will mostly be effective at making people feel bad about their lives and electing terrible presidents, but the one good thing that will come of it is that you will see this day for what it was and see yourself for what you were: beautiful and happy."

I'd also tell her that she was never going to win a best actress Oscar so she should just let that one go and get on with her life.

Casa Diablo:

In Which a Stripper's Vagina and a Blind Chihuahua Cause Me to Send a Monumental Text

My friend Rich needed someone to help him entertain his uncle.

That's how I got a vagina in my face.

Rich is what I call a "wide-net flirter." Wide-net flirters work their charms on anything with a pulse for two reasons: One, they never know when their scattershot advances will magically find purchase with a big-league hottie, and two, even if they're not attracted to the objects of their random affection, they almost always get attention in return.

Rich and I had been hanging out for about a year and a half with a large group of friends. He had flirted with me from the very beginning, which was shocking to me because I weighed two hundred and forty pounds and being flirted with was a real anomaly. In my experience, when you weigh two hundred and forty pounds, most men actively avoid your gaze just in case you're the type of girl who mistakes eye contact for attraction. Relative invisibility—just part of the fun of being fat.[1]

Rich was a short man with a big personality—he was charismatic and smart with bright, impish brown eyes and a nice, juicy sense of humor. At parties he'd smile at me a lot, wait a noticeably long time to break eye contact, and usually find a way to inject a little sexual innuendo into every conversation, even when it was a bit of a stretch: "Yeah, Iran should withdraw their troops. I always retreat before my advances result in a long-term engagement."

Because it'd been a long time since anyone flirted with me, I made the mistake of taking Rich seriously and imagined that, at some point, our flirtation would lead somewhere. And it did lead somewhere: a trip to Casa Diablo, the world's first vegan strip club.

When he asked me to go, it seemed like the perfect outing for my project. I'd heard that the strippers at Casa Diablo were pretty aggressive, and the phrase *aggressive strippers* made me wince just enough to put this idea at about a 7 on the Uneasiness Scale. Plus, I liked spending time with Rich and thought this would be a great way to show him what a super-fun, no-sexual-hang-ups kinda lady I was, so I joined him.

Just to be clear, I wasn't totally subjugating myself to a man's whims on the off chance that it might lead to a make-out session. I've done that in the past, sure, but not this time. I had been to,

---

1   Other fun things about being fat include, but are not limited to, walking down a plane aisle and watching people cringe as you approach; clothing with giant floral patterns that make one appear couch-y; and random men on the street saying things like "Wow. Look at that ass. I know you can cook. I'll marry you." See? Fun.

and somewhat uncomfortably enjoyed, strip clubs before. I believe that what strippers do on the pole is unquestionably an art form and should be under consideration as an Olympic sport. It would bring in an entirely new demographic, and TV ratings would skyrocket. Other suggestions for Olympic sports: Butt-Plug Shotput, Stiletto Balance Beam, and General Thong Tolerance. I'm just spitballing here.

Case Diablo stood alone on a hill on Highway 30 in Portland, an industrial road right across from a train yard on the Willamette River. The building looked like it used to be a faux Western saloon, with a wooden facade and a huge porch that ran the length of the building. Prior to being a strip club, it was a nautically themed vegan restaurant called Pirates' Tavern Grub and Grog. I'd eaten there years before, when a friend went to review it. It looked different now.

A middle-aged, slightly rough-around-the-edges woman sat at a table at the entrance with a cash box in front of her.

"It's five bucks to get in," she said. "For an extra two dollars, you can see my tits."

I wanted the whole experience so I splurged for the bonus boobs.

She took my money, then unceremoniously flopped out her left breast before making change for other customers. I'm not sure what I thought two dollars would get me, but it was more than that.

"Thanks!" I crooned sweetly as I entered. Because manners are important.

The club still looked a bit like a diner, with booths lining one wall in the front, but it was dark, and we were surrounded by barebreasted and heavily tatted women walking adeptly on seven-inch heels while balancing trays of french fries and cocktails.

There were no longer tables in the center of the long space; they'd been replaced by a stage that extended almost the full length of the club. It was split into thirds lengthwise, and each section had its own pole you could sit close to at the rack (the front-row seat) if you were brave enough. It was theater-in-the-round but with butts and vaginas and stuff.

If you wanted to sit at the rack, you had to put a two-dollar bill in front of you for every song, so we went to get our stack of twos from one of the bartenders, all of whom were also topless. In the same way I find Halloween disconcerting (*Is it fun or appalling that my urgent-care nurse has a witch's nose on right now?*), I found it strange to have a topless woman doing things like making change and flipping a cocktail shaker. It was like the old *Playgirl* centerfolds where the photographer had apparently caught the oiled-up hunk fixing an old Chevy or fishing with his "tackle out," so to speak—the scene was supposed to be sexy just because the guy happened to be naked. But for me, nude oil changes and typing drink orders into a tablet aren't sexy. Sex acts are sexy.

I knew my reaction was unusual, especially since every one of the women in Casa Diablo was stunning. The majority of them were in the SuicideGirls vein—elaborate, artistic tattoos, Bettie Page haircuts, and perfectly toned, healthy bodies. All of which sent me into a complex mental cat's cradle of assertions and rationalizations.

ME: Jesus, they're gorgeous.

FEMINIST BUZZKILL ME: You don't get to decide they're gorgeous. What's *gorgeous* anyway? Muscular and tiny? Fuck you.

ME: Well, I live in our culture, so yes, I've been socialized to think that. And gorgeous isn't a bad thing.

FBM: You're objectifying them.

ME: But they should be able to do whatever they want with their bodies.

FBM: Right, but they're being judged by everyone here, so the power dynamic that should tip in their favor tips the other way. In most of these people's minds, they're sluts.

ME: Yeah, but the actual power dynamic is that men leave their homes and sit literally dumbstruck, dropping hundreds of dollars, while women they're not allowed to touch shake their hips a bit in front of them and maybe get on their laps. If aliens landed and saw this dynamic, they'd think women were worshipped as gods. Which they kind of are.

FBM: Gods who make eighty cents on the dollar, you mean?

ME: Jesus, you are horrible to hang out with.

It is exhausting for me to go out with me.

My internal dialogue was interrupted by the screeching announcer's voice over the loudspeaker.

"And now, coming to the stage, a girl whose pussy will make you purr! Give it up for the best tail in the house—Miss Kitty!"

Jesus Christ.

Rich and I sat down at the front end of the rack and slapped one of our two-dollar bills on the table. Kitty came out in a bra and underwear, as strippers are wont to do, and was less enthused about dancing than about making the pole her shiny metal bitch. At one point she climbed to the ceiling on the pole (not an easy feat when you're slathered in glitter lotion and wearing seven-inch heels), scissored her straightened legs around it, and hung there, her body perfectly perpendicular to the pole. Then she spun, still in that position, all the way down to the stage. I was mesmerized. I also wondered if OSHA spent a lot of time here checking poles for structural integrity.

At such moments, most audience members are imagining what it would be like to be that pole and have that much power wrapped around them. But I was thinking about whether the cleaner they used on the pole between dancers might cause a rash.

My imagination falls short with anything involving strip clubs. This seems to run in my family. My brother, Scott, once told me about a trip he'd taken to Mexico with a friend of his who wanted to visit a prostitute. Scott agreed at first but couldn't go through with it.

"I couldn't suspend my disbelief," he said.

I had the same problem with porn. When I did watch it—I have been single for the majority of my adult life and have often needed assistance with fantasizing—I discovered that it was really difficult for me to be turned on if the actors were bad and the women weren't actually aroused. Not a lot of Yale Drama grads in porn, and most women don't have orgasms from penetration alone, so it was hard for me to find effective porn (#firstworldproblems).

So I wasn't turned on yet at the strip club, but I did learn something useful for my next bachelorette party: bejeweled anal plugs are a thing.

At one point, the second stripper, whose vaguely morning-show-esque face caused us to dub her "Kelly Ripa's Alternate Timeline," was spinning around the pole, ass akimbo, and I saw something shiny between her...cheeks. It looked like a two-inch-wide diamond. So if you were thinking that innovations in the lucrative world of taking off one's clothes had ceased, you were dead wrong.

I knew I was being rude to Kelly, but I just had to do a cursory internet search on my phone and it brought up Swarovski Crystal Jeweled Butt Plugs, which, the website boasted, "make anal play even more fun by adding glamour and bling." (I thought anal play was already glamorous enough. I stood corrected.)

My inability to suspend my disbelief reared its ugly head once again when Scarlett, the third dancer, approached me. She was completely naked save for her almost-full-body floral tattoos,[2] and she came to sit at the edge of the rack in front of me. She wrapped her legs around my arms, and her hands explored my body. All I could feel was a wave of red washing over my face and neck.

"Cute outfit," she whispered sweetly into my ear, her breasts three inches from my face.

It was like I was sort of at a strip club but also sort of at brunch.

"Thanks?" I replied, thinking I should return the compliment. *Cute vagina?*

I decided not to say anything and just smiled, glanced over at Rich, and "laughed." (*Ohmigod, could I be more fun or easygoing? No!*) In retrospect, I think my expression probably looked more like a grimace.

Next, Scarlett lay down on her back, wrapped her legs around my neck, and pulled my face closer and closer to the aforementioned

---

2   Strippers in Oregon can be completely naked due to a 2005 Oregon Supreme Court decision that declared that nude dancing was protected under the state constitution's free-speech provisions. There are so many ways to express yourself in Oregon. Naked is just one of them.

cute, hairless vagina until it was inches away. I'd never seen another vagina in person, at least from this angle and proximity.

Like the snowflakes of the genital world, no two vaginas are alike. Hers had tiny labia majora (the outer lips) and larger labia minora (the inside, more Georgia O'Keeffe–style lips). She had minor majoras and major minoras, is what I'm saying.

This might not be relevant to the story. Apologies.

Before I even had time to register all the details of her Lady Snowflake, she was grinding on my lap with her hands running through my hair and my face between her breasts.

Score! Right?

Here's what went through my head: *I just washed this skirt, and now there's stranger vagina all over it.*

I generally like having naked genitals grinding on me, but it's usually prefaced by some drinks, a lot of flirting, and a conversation in which I can get a feel for someone's political affiliation. Also, the genitals I enjoy are usually penis-and-ball-shaped, but why get technical?

Rich laughed the whole time, which was an appropriate response given the fact that I was fake-laughing.

What am I doing? Why can't I just apologize to Scarlett for not fully appreciating her vagina and get up and leave?

Like many women, I've spent a lot of time in my life enduring subtly uncomfortable situations in order to avoid overtly uncomfortable situations.

Scarlett would've probably been mildly offended, and Rich would've realized that I wasn't the breezy, up-for-anything gal-about-town I was pretending to be, but at least it would've been over more quickly.

Thankfully, "Pour Some Sugar on Me" ended and Scarlett left to crawl around the stage picking up her tips, taking her vagina with her. Buzzkill Me screamed, *See? She's literally crawling on the stage for her money!* while postmodern, third-wave-feminist, pro-porn me shook her head and held up a white flag.

I thought about why I was there.

I'm shattering my comfort zone, right? I have a column to write. This will make a great story.

I was full of shit.

I *was* subjugating myself to Rich's whims. And at a strip club, no less, where subjugating women was the *whole point.*

By the time we finally left, I felt far dirtier for pretending to be chill than I did for watching naked women gyrate all night.

At the Casa Diablo point in my bizarre friendship-with-no-discernible-benefits relationship with Rich, I'd lost over sixty pounds and was no longer the two-hundred-forty-pound unhappy person I'd been when we first met.

A few months prior, I'd had a gallbladder attack and had it removed. I was told to eat a strict low-fat diet, which I did for fear of the consequences if I didn't. (Fun body fact: Your gallbladder sends additional bile to your stomach to help you digest when you eat a lot of fat, so if you don't have a gallbladder, your body can sometimes say WTF? in really gross ways if you eat fries.) Turned out that one of the few things that could motivate me to lose weight was a constant, nagging fear of death that began when I spent a few hours in the hospital waiting room pre-surgery thinking I was having a heart attack. Not recommended, but effective as hell.

So, more than sixty pounds down, I was feeling pretty good about myself. And yet I was still having difficulty imagining that there were other men besides Rich who might be attracted to me. Once you internalize fat-shaming, even when you lose weight, your brain's muscle memory keeps snapping back to "I am unlovable." I was a healthy size 16 who worked out like a fiend, but my brain was still a size 24 with high blood pressure.

In the weeks after Casa Diablo, I spent a couple of nights at Rich's after attending parties at his house because I was "way too drunk to go home,"[3] and he never touched me.

In fact, the second time I spent the night in his bed, he told me that I shouldn't sleep in my clothes because "Who does that?" I agreed that clothes were dumb,[4] and because his comment seemed like a precursor to the sex I was hoping to have, I took mine off and got back in bed.

I lay there expectantly, listening to his breathing to see if he was sleeping and trying to decipher with each movement whether he was moving closer to me. It was a king-size bed, so it was hard to tell.

Nothing happened.

Well, something happened; it just wasn't sex. In an insult-to-injury situation, after about thirty minutes of lying in silence, Rich proceeded to place his old Chihuahua between us on the bed, just to ensure that I couldn't possibly touch him.

I was cockblocked by a tiny blind Chihuahua.

---

3 I wasn't.
4 They're not.

I lay there for a while pondering the fact that Rich had used his lapdog as a sex barricade, then slithered silently out of his bed, got dressed, and went downstairs to sleep on the couch.

The next morning he asked why I left his bed.

"Did I snore?" he said, grinning.

No, I was just having trouble breathing through the impenetrable fog of humiliation.

"Yes," I responded. "And so did your dog."

After every interaction with him, I told myself I had to stop hoping, but then the next interaction happened, and my hope would rear its head again.

Just a couple months after the Chihuahua Incident, on New Year's Eve, Rich and I found ourselves facing each other in a crowded room at a party thrown by mutual friends. Once again, I imagined there was a chance we'd end up making out in a closet somewhere. (What is it about romantic possibility that can turn a lifelong pessimist into an optimist?) The night was filled with knowing glances and too-long hugs, but nothing else.

The next morning, I was done.

Things are always clearer in the morning, but they're particularly clear on New Year's Day, when you're taking a good, hard look at your life, or at least as good a look as you can get while painfully squinting through sunglasses. So I decided I'd lay everything out on the table with Rich once and for all.

After a hungover breakfast with friends, I pulled out my phone to call him.

Instead, I opened up sudoku.

I played for half an hour.

I checked my e-mail. No one but Bed, Bath, and Beyond was e-mailing me on New Year's Day.

I thought about whether new hand towels would make this a better year for me.

I checked Facebook. I looked at what felt like hundreds of pictures of friends in wacky hats, kissing each other.

Fucking New Year's Eve.

I'm calling him.

I went to dial.

I wasn't going to call him.

The problem was, I am of the WASP people, and we are so averse to confrontation that we would sooner crawl into a dragon's gaping, steaming asshole than tell a waiter our hamburgers are overcooked.

I decided to go the coward's route. I texted him.

Hey! Weird text: I just want to clarify something—you seem sort of attracted to me, but not quite enough to ever fuck me or date me. Does that seem accurate? I know it's awkward but I just need to know definitively because it's always felt like there was an energy between us but I think it's just an energy you have with all women. Don't feel bad either way. It'd just be a relief to know it'll never actually go anywhere.

It was a really long text.

I waited for his response. The three little dots appeared, indicating he was typing. I swallowed hard.

I already felt so dumb.

I'd spent over a year wondering if anything would ever happen with this guy, deconstructing our texts and interactions with friends like a teenager wondering if a boy was going to ask her to go steady. I'd spent an hour naked in bed while an old blind Chihuahua snored on my boobs. And I'd spent one strange evening with what seemed like a very nice woman's genitals in my face.

When you invest that much energy in someone, it's daunting to ask a question whose answer has the capacity to turn you into the world's biggest fool.

I regretted not having gotten a bloody mary with my eggs.

Finally, his response:

I'm so flattered, and I definitely have a crush on you and have a lot of fun flirting, but you're one of my favorite people in the world and I'd never want to ruin that with any sex stuff. I do that with most women and their always ending up mad at me. We should talk about this in person, though.

Translation: *I'm not as attracted to you as you are to me and, oops, sorry about all the flirting that I knew wasn't going anywhere, but who takes that shit seriously? What're you, twelve? Also, let's meet so I can look you in the eye while you talk about how attracted you are to me.*

The fog of humiliation rolled in again. I took a deep breath.

How could I ever have liked someone who didn't know the difference between *they're* and *their*?

It was just so ridiculous, and more than a little sad. I had been so grateful to him for paying attention to me that I had somehow not noticed that other men had started doing the same thing. I'd lost all that physical weight, but clearly I was still carrying around some of the metaphorical variety.

Plus, I didn't have a lot of practical experience with men. I'd had two short relationships since I was in high school, so of course I was acting like a teenager—when it came to romantic love, I was one.

I had to remedy that.

I felt so behind—I was in my forties and all my friends had had plenty of relationships by now. The bad boys, the good ones you let get away because you weren't good yet, the sweet-yet-sad one, the one who brought out the worst in you, the one you hurt, the one who really knew how to hurt you, the one who taught you to speak up for yourself, the uppity "healthy-lifestyle" one that just made you want to drink more bourbon, the one who blinded you with that one cool thing he did so you couldn't see he was a total asshole.

And, of course, the heart-wrenching one where you were still in love but the other person just ran out of it like it was milk or eggs, and you thought, *But those are* staples. *You pay attention, and you always replenish the staples.*

I'd at least had that one.

Even so, I knew when it came to relationships, I was the personification of Donald Rumsfeld's "unknown unknowns"—there were so many things I didn't know, I didn't even know I didn't know them yet.

That's when I decided to add dating to the OFW Project.

I had never dated in my life. The two people I'd had relationships with, I'd met through friends, and we went immediately from being friends to being "together."

I was going to sign up for a dating site. And I was going to...date people. Strangers, even.

The thought of it created a tiny new dread ball, but I knew I had to muster the courage to address this thing head-on, much like I'd addressed the vagina in my face a few months earlier.

It was time. I was ready.

I was nauseated.

I fixed a bloody mary and downloaded the OkCupid app.

A Little Bit of Background:

Wherein I Attempt to Explain My Dating Situation

It may be difficult for you to understand why, at forty-five years old, I had the relationship experience of a twenty-one-year-old.

It is also difficult for me to understand.

I think I can trace at least some of it back to a moment when I was sixteen.

I'd always been slightly heavier than my friends, but that year, my father was pressuring me to transfer to a private school and after five moves in my lifetime the idea of yet another school was overwhelming. I really started overachieving in the overeating department.

We were living in Salinas, California, at the time, in a house with a basement bedroom that my brother, Scott, lived in. He took great advantage of having a separate entrance—he always had a girlfriend or three, some of whom we met and some of whom we just heard through the screen door, whispering expletives as they snagged their jeans on the blackberry bushes while sneaking out at midnight.

His room was under our dining room, and the heating vent on the dining-room floor went directly through to his ceiling.

One night, two of his friends, Shawn and Dave, slept over. I had a crush on Shawn because his hair looked like a shorter version of Eddie Van Halen's and he wore his T-shirts so small that the sleeves always seemed greatly taxed by his muscles. I decided to listen in on their conversation in case Shawn said anything about me.

It was after midnight, and my parents were already asleep.

I walked quietly out of my bedroom and past my parents' room to the living room. Even though we had carpeting, I knew Scott could still hear every footfall, so, in an attempt to evenly distribute my weight and cause fewer creaks, I got down on my hands and knees and crawled across the living-room floor. I heard the boys' muffled voices rise up through the vent from ten feet away.

The vent was long, slim, and metal, the kind with slats pointing in opposite directions from the middle. I laid my ear on it and felt the cold metal digging into my cheek. Shawn was talking.

"Shut up, man," he said. "She likes you and you know it. They all like you."

"They do not," Dave said. "Just, like . . . I don't know . . . most of them."

They all laughed.

Dave was blond and built like a football player. All the girls did like him.

"You're such an asshole," Scott said.

"Oh, I'm the asshole?" Dave said. "What about you? How many girlfriends do you have right now?"

"Both of you need to shut up," said Shawn. "It's depressing."

I drew in a breath and held it, listening for any word that might pertain to me.

"Aw, you're fine, man," Dave said. "I heard Dana Mitchell likes you."

"Dana?" Shawn said. "Seriously? Why is it that only the fat girls like me?"

"I don't know," Dave said. "Maybe because you look really delicious?"

Uproarious laughter bounced up through the vent and echoed into my ear. I sat up, the indentations of the vent slats still in my cheek.

I was fatter than Dana Mitchell.

I leaned against the wall, hugging my knees, deciding at that moment that I would never be the fat girl who likes the boy who doesn't like her back.

So there may have been many times in my life when men expressed an interest in me, but I was too busy projecting the idea that I didn't like anyone, ever, to see that interest. And that projection may have made me appear at times somewhat unwelcoming or, quite literally, impenetrable.

And then when I was thirty-four, I lost seventy-five pounds.[1]

And just like what happened a decade later, suddenly I didn't feel like the vulnerable big girl who couldn't express an interest in anyone. I felt almost standard size, and in my mind, standard-size women

---

1 "But wait," you might say. "Didn't you lose sixty pounds a decade later, right before the Casa Diablo debacle?" I did. But it was sixty of the seventy-five pounds that I had regained over the previous decade. That's how weight works: like a wildly ineffective, never-ending treadmill.

were free to let men know they were interested without (as much) fear of being laughed at.

That's when I met the first person I ever fell in love with.

He was the owner of a vintage-camera-and-typewriter store in Portland. The night we met, I was sitting at a bar patio with a large group and noticed him at one of our shared picnic tables talking to my friend Matt. He was wearing jeans and old boots and a beat-up vintage-leather field jacket over a white T-shirt. His thick, light brown hair arced up and flopped charmingly onto his forehead in a very "Robert Redford in *The Way We Were*" kind of way and he was gesticulating wildly as he spoke. He had the brightest blue eyes I'd ever seen.

Matt introduced us and we talked for an hour. His name was Jake and he told me that if I put the right typewriter on a big metal desk, my writing could sound like an oncoming train. He was charming and strange and passionate about beautiful, obsolete machines, which might have been why he was attracted to me.

We went on a date a week later to see a jug band a work acquaintance of his was in. Even in the throes of insane attraction, it's difficult to act interested in jug-band music, but I did.

"I'm so sorry," he said when it was over. "That may have been the worst thing I've ever done to anyone."

I laughed.

"It was fine," I said.

"It was like some ancient form of hillbilly torture," he said. "I'm never going to see you again, am I?"

"You will," I said. "But I'll be asking you to accompany me to listen to some dental drills and a circular saw played in an abandoned mental institution."

"Sounds fair," he said.

He asked if I wanted to come back to his place in St. Johns, an older neighborhood in North Portland, for a nightcap. I nodded and speed-walked to my car to follow him home.

We walked through the entryway into a living room that he clearly hadn't really been living in. Beautiful dark hardwood floors, a fireplace, a long window seat, and just one item: a vintage record player in the corner. Jake explained that his ex had left a few months prior and he hadn't gotten around to replacing any of their stuff.

"You wanna come upstairs to the attic and see my typewriters?" he asked.

"Really? Does that work on people?"

"I think it's about to work on you." He grinned.

It did.

Long before I ever met him, I'd been collecting old cameras and typewriters, so it was as if his whole house and store and body and brain were all elaborate traps built especially for me.[2]

He asked me if I wanted a glass of red wine. I said yes. I hated red wine, but I had a plan.

See, I was a virgin, and I wanted desperately to get rid of that albatross that was hanging around my . . . vagina. It had turned me into a total freak, this virginity I couldn't seem to get rid of. I skirted around the issue with him, saying things like "When it comes to dating, just consider me a sort of tabula rasa" and "I've never really been the dat-

---

2   It may appear that he was a hipster poseur, but remember that this was the early aughts, so it was way before the rest of the world became fascinated with typewriters, retro iPhone filters, and vinyl.

ing type. I'm more of a let's-hang-out-and-see-what-happens type." I thought if we got totally wasted, we could just do it and get it over with and it would be this teeny lie of omission.

I wasn't thinking about what it would be like the next morning or the fact that I actually liked this guy and kicking off a physical relationship with him with a lie was maybe a bad idea, not to mention borderline evil. But when you're thirty-four and an accidental virgin, desperation can cloud your judgment.

We took the wine upstairs and he opened up a door on his giant old metal desk and pulled out a shelf that housed a shiny, sleek 1960s-era burgundy Smith Corona portable that looked like a sports car. He had me sit down and type on it, and it was the sexiest foreplay to foreplay I'd ever experienced.

But it turned out there wasn't going to be any actual foreplay that night. I did sleep over, but in my shirt and a pair of his pajama bottoms that did not look cute on me. And nothing happened.

I awoke the next morning when I heard him stir. As we both ungroggified ourselves, we chatted about important subjects like how we slept and what kind of sheets he had. Then, as he was brushing his teeth in the bathroom, we continued an earlier conversation about our dating histories.

I don't remember what I said to stop him in his tracks; I just remember that at some point, I no longer heard the *whoosh-whoosh-whoosh* of him brushing his teeth, and then he showed up in his bedroom doorway holding his toothbrush and looking both shocked and entertained.

"You're a *virshin!*" he yelled toothpastily.

Yes, damn it. I was a virshin.

I'd thought I could avoid it, but I had to tell him. Mostly because I liked him, but also because I'm not evil. Mostly.

"I am," I said. "But it's not on purpose, I promise. I really *want* to have sex, it's just that the opportunity hasn't arisen yet, or when it did arise, I didn't take it because I thought it would arise again and then it kind of didn't."

Well, that didn't sound good. The last thing you want to hear about someone you're interested in is that no one else wanted her. People are always questioning their judgment at the beginning of a relationship, and what I'd just said was exhibit A in the case for "This is a shut-in/loser/psychopath and I should run away right now even though my mouth is full of toothpaste and this is my house."

I could've attempted to come up with an excuse.

Sex was forbidden in the nunnery. And technically I'm still married. To God.

Or *I could've had sex, but I was in a state of suspended animation in space for fifteen years. When I woke up, we had to battle this giant bug-like alien with acid spit. It was terrible.*

Or simply *I'm Canadian.*

But none of those would've made any difference. He went and spat out his toothpaste and came and sat next to me on his bed.

"So, I really like you. A lot," he said, lowering his head to make sure he caught my eye.

I knew where this was going and my stomach already hurt.

"But...I just don't think I can take this on," he said.

"Yeah. I get it."

"I'd really like to be your friend, though," he continued.

I hadn't been looking to make any friends whose bones I constantly wanted to jump but wasn't allowed to, so this wasn't great news.

"Sounds good," I said.

I could've argued with him, I suppose, told him I was worth his getting past the pain-in-the-ass-ness of the situation, but I wasn't sure I was. I understood his fear because I had it myself. By the time most people are thirty-four, they've had multiple relationships and they've learned all the important lessons about how to fight without throwing things, what their deal breakers are, and what fetishes they can tolerate/might actually enjoy.

I was already so behind.

I sat staring at his blank bedroom wall, knowing this conversation was probably going to keep happening with every man I met.

He brought me tea and toast with jam in bed and we talked for a while before going up to the attic to hang out. As "friends."

I felt sad and more than a little rejected, but it didn't take long for me to get sucked into my surroundings. The attic was surprisingly warm and cozy, with crisscross-paned windows and old filing cabinets topped with vintage wire in-boxes that held stacks of paper I wanted to snoop through.

We talked and he showed me some of the black-and-white portraits he'd taken of his friends (none of them were naked, which made me relieved that he wasn't "that guy"). Then he put on a Tom Waits CD and read and napped on an old couch next to the desk while I typed on his Underwood (note: not a euphemism).

It felt like a perfect afternoon.

And then, because it was so perfect, it couldn't have been more imperfect.

This was what I would be missing because I had this fucking vaginal albatross.

"I'm gonna go, I think," I said, waking him up.

"Oh. Okay," he said, looking at his watch. It was about four in the afternoon. "You sure you don't want to stay for supper?"

Yes. It's everything I want, actually. Everything.

"No. I'm good. I just need to go."

We went downstairs and I put on my tights and shoes in his bedroom, the same spot where I'd had so much hope just a few hours prior.

Stupid bedroom.

He walked me to his entryway and opened the front door.

"Well, I had a great time," he said.

"Yeah, it was really nice. Thanks so much for breakfast and for the drinks."

"Of course," he said. "Are you sure you don't want to stay? I could cook some pork chops."

"No, but thank you." I just wanted out of there. I thought I might cry and I didn't want him to see that. (*Hey, remember when you thought you shouldn't date me because what kind of freak is a virgin at thirty-four? How 'bout the kind of freak who cries after a first date?*)

"Can I at least hug you good-bye?" he asked.

"Of course you can," I said.

He went in for a hug but kissed me instead.

He kissed me so hard, it threw both of our bodies up against the wall in his entryway, his chest pressing into mine and every limb I could spare pulling him in with equal force. My hands were immediately in his hair and tugging at his shirt. I finally understood what people meant when they said they wanted to devour someone. I'd never been hungrier.

After about five minutes of this, he finally came up for air and stepped back. He looked like a feral animal. In a good way.

I attempted to recombobulate myself.

"Well. All right," I said.

"Uh-huh," he replied. "So, yeah. So you should stay for dinner. We can make out more."

I wanted so much to stay. But the problem was that it wasn't all I wanted. I didn't want to just make out with this person, I wanted to stay with him and then wake up with him. Multiple times, ideally. Maybe all the times.

"I think I'm gonna go," I heard myself say.

"Really?" he said.

"Yeah," I said. "You're ambivalent about me, I think. So I'm gonna go, and you can think about all this and figure out where you stand."

He seemed genuinely shocked.

"Okay," he said. "I guess I'll do that."

"Okay," I said, and I smiled as I walked out.

It was by far the coolest thing I'd ever done.

And even before I got off the porch, I regretted it. All I could think in my car on the way home was *What did I just do?*

I thought I'd made the biggest mistake of my life. Until he called three days later. He wanted to cook me dinner, and I accepted. Which also had the potential to be the biggest mistake of my life.

A week later, he made me pork chops and we fell in love.

It took him three months to finally take my albatross, and because he'd spent that time figuring out what I liked, and I'd spent even longer reading a great book called *The Guide to Getting It On,* a huge eight-hundred-page tome with chapters like "The Glands Down Under" and "Fun with Your Foreskin," it was actually quite lovely.

I felt very lucky about that. After waiting as long as I had, it would've been horrible if it had been horrible. Which is probably why he didn't want the pressure in the first place.

Once I'd had sex, I wanted to have it *all the time.* And we did. In fact, if you lived in the greater Portland area between August of 2002 and April of 2004 and you noticed a slight downturn in the sexual activity in your relationship...we were probably having your sex too. Which I'd like to apologize for. But I won't take it back. Believe me, the world owed me that sex.

And I guess with all that doin' it, I was distracted from the fact that I was making the classic rookie mistake: As I fell into him, I fell away from myself, almost completely. I was so grateful to him for loving me that I was perfectly happy to step into his life and leave mine behind. I hosted his cocktail parties, hung out with his friends...I even took on his temperament. I thought my goofiness wasn't very sexy, so, for the most part, I ditched it.

I loved to chat, but he was careful with his words. I would hunt for topics that he'd think were interesting. At the end of the day, I mostly wanted to talk about my job and my friends, but I could tell he didn't find those subjects compelling, so I'd try to work those stories into a larger context.

"Looks like Karen's getting divorced," I'd say. "People keep saying that divorce rates are skyrocketing, but in fact, they've been steadily declining for the past decade. Isn't that weird?"

It was fucking exhausting.

I envy the reticent. They hold so much power.

I would ramble on and on while he sat and listened and judged.

Or at least it felt like judgment.

It was probably just boredom.

That's just as bad. Maybe worse? Hard to decide.

I used to think that in order to seem smart and interesting, I needed to reveal all the things about me that were smart and interesting in conversation. But I learned the hard way that the more I revealed about myself, the less interesting I became. At least to him.

He was a goddamn sphinx, so of course I still found him fascinating.

And even though the conversation didn't always flow, I still thought I was happy.

I was loved. Right?

Lots of things suggested we weren't right for each other, but other things suggested we should hunker down and work it out.

He could be incredibly sweet.

One night we were on the couch in front of a raging fire. He was reading a Michael Chabon novel and I was working on a sketch for the show. He was sitting sideways with his feet toward me, sometimes rubbing my leg to get my attention, like a Labrador. I would rub his foot for a minute and we'd lock eyes and smile and then go back to our respective book and laptop.

The next morning as we were waking up, he said, "Last night? Sitting on the couch reading while you wrote? That was perfect. Thank you for making my life into exactly what I want it to be."

But over time, he became increasingly frustrated with my neuroses, as did I. Neither of us knew that I had generalized anxiety disorder.

One night as I was lying in his bed reading, he walked in and told me that he had noticed a small growth on my back.

"Really?" I said, immediately reaching over to feel it.

"Calm down," he said. "I'm not gonna break up with you because you have a fucking mole."

I was always nervous about our relationship, so he wasn't totally off base, but in that case I wasn't worried he would break up with me, I was immediately sure I had skin cancer and would die within a year, so I was thinking about what countries I should travel to.

So we were already on shaky ground when it finally cracked beneath us.

Our friend Josey died in May of 2004. She was just a few days shy of her thirtieth birthday.

Really, she was Jake's friend. He'd brought her to Portland to work with him in his camera store. Josey was one of an army of fiercely loyal minions he had. They were people who believed in the power of old machines and the permanence of photo paper. They were anti-digital, anti–planned obsolescence, and pro–art that is very, very labor-intensive to create.

I'd been dating Jake for two years and had grown to love Josey. She was impossible not to love and as different from Jake as she could be. He would walk to the store from his home close by, dressed in khakis, a sweater vest, and a tie. Josey rode a Razor Scooter with a monkey head on the handlebars, and she'd once paired a set of human-size butterfly wings with purple Doc Martens for a store party. When customers walked into the store, Jake would look up from his work and give them the Nod. Josey would run around the counter to give them rib-cracking bear hugs. She was the heart of that place, and in some ways I imagined she was his heart. Jake cared strongly about his customers and friends but his introversion didn't allow him to run around the counter to hug them. Josey was his hugger-by-proxy.

Their relationship was both professional and personal—Josey was a badass, do-whatever-it-takes-to-get-the-job-done employee and also the little sister that he (an only child) had never had.

On May 8, 2004, Josey left Portland to drive to her parents' house in Port Orchard, Washington, to celebrate Mother's Day and her birthday.

Jake's phone rang at three a.m.

She was only about forty miles outside of Portland on I-5 North when she hydroplaned and her car spun around and landed next to the median, backward. She got out of the car, perhaps to open up the hood to indicate she needed help, and another car hydroplaned in the exact same spot, spun, and hit her, throwing her about twenty feet onto the pavement.

We wouldn't know it for about three weeks, but for all intents and purposes, Josey died that night.

Her parents, Randy and Marion, drove down from Port Orchard as soon as they got the call.

I drove Jake to the hospital at three a.m. I spent about four hours in the waiting room while it started to get light outside. Jake emerged at about seven thirty a.m., and we walked out into the cool May air, the grass on the front lawn still dewy with mist from the night before. His face looked drained and blank as he matter-of-factly told me what had happened to her.

It was bad. She'd lost her legs, aspirated fluid into her lungs, and been put into a medically induced coma.

He broke down, and I let him fall into me, sobbing.

It was Mother's Day.

I took Randy and Marion back to Jake's house to get them settled in. Jake wouldn't leave the hospital. He slept in the fetal position on a tiny couch outside the ICU that night, with one of those scratchy, too-small blankets that make everyone look like a child. He didn't leave that couch for three weeks.

As Josey's body fought to survive, her friends and family filed into the hospital, one by one and in groups, reading three-year-old magazines over and over again and talking about mundane things to avoid talking about devastating, life-altering, heartbreaking things.

Jake's mother flew in that first week to help but only after he very pointedly told her, "If you come, you can't be my mother. I need a driver, a shopper, a bed-maker, and a phone-call-maker. That's the kind of help I need."

What he was saying to her but never said to me was *Don't love me. Don't touch me. Don't comfort me. It will break me.*

He was taking care of everything, dealing with the police and the hospital and insurance companies, and he believed, I think, that if he took any kindness, leaned in to a warm shoulder or returned a sympathetic glance, it would weaken him and he would never recover.

I spent those weeks helping take care of the out-of-town guests, doing the grocery shopping and cooking meals, making beds and taxiing people between the hospital and Jake's house. I was shell-shocked and sad, watching this extraordinary couple as their daughter slipped away from the world while at the same time watching Jake slip away from me.

He would give me my assignments and then offer a perfunctory hug, but other than that, this previously affectionate (to me) person became cold and businesslike. He would sit as far from me as possible in the hospital waiting room. When I touched him, he would cringe and turn away.

On May 28, 2004, three weeks after the accident, Josey died.

The funeral was a week later in Port Orchard, Washington, about a three-hour drive from Portland. Jake and I drove up in a rental car along with a couple other friends and stayed in Josey's old house with her parents. We were given the guest room—a perfect 1970s semifinished basement room with shag carpeting and a yellow floral bedspread.

Jake was still emotionally distant but was at least holding me as we slept, which was perhaps my favorite part of dating him. Every night we spent together, as we prepared to go to sleep, he would wrap both his arms around me and pull me in as tightly as possible, the way you tie your boots before a long hike. It was as if he didn't want a millimeter of space between us. It made me feel loved and safe, and most of the time it made me forget whatever perceived crimes of his I'd shoved all the way down into the dark recesses of my subconscious that day.

After Josey died, Jake had let me know that Kelley, his ex-girlfriend of eleven years, would be attending the funeral. They'd broken up just five months before he and I started dating and he was understandably concerned about my feelings. I appreciated it but told him I was looking forward to meeting her. I wasn't, but that's just one of those things you say to not sound nuts.

The funeral was at Marion and Randy's Lutheran church, the same church that Josey had attended as a kid. It was beautiful and poignant and filled with hundreds of people trying to make sense of the utterly senseless.

After the funeral, there was a potluck where we all ate way too many carbs and milled around for about an hour, until it was time to head over to the grave site for the interment. People started getting into their cars. I looked around, but Jake had disappeared. I asked Zeb, who worked in the store with Jake, if he knew where he was, and he told me he thought he'd seen him with Kelley. I looked out the back door of the church and saw the two of them walking away into the woods. There were a few of us going in the same car, so we waited for them.

We sat in the back hallway of the church making small talk as more time passed. Fifteen minutes. Then twenty-five minutes. Then thirty. We were all fine at the beginning of this waiting period, but after a while, things got uncomfortable. I started having a hard time with the fact that my boyfriend had disappeared with his ex-girlfriend for a half an hour without saying a word to me. Of course I didn't think anything illicit was happening between them. I wasn't crazy enough to picture them having postfuneral sex in the woods. I was just feeling like...an asshole. Like the person who, along with a whole passel of other supportive people, had seen this man through a life-shattering experience and was now being treated just a little like shit.

I knew my feelings were ill timed, but there they were, bubbling up and then bubbling over and slathering every good intention I had in black, tarlike emotional bile. Maybe being angry felt more comfortable than being sad.

We finally decided not to wait anymore and walked out to the church parking lot, and that's when Jake and Kelley showed up. When Jake spoke to me, I don't remember what I said, but I do remember that I was a bitch. I was short with both him and Kelley and couldn't look either of them in the eye. We got into the car and drove to the grave site.

The spot where Josey was interred was beautiful—a perfect, tiny but lush knoll under a big shady tree.

As Jake and I stood next to the grave, he put his arm around me. I was sobbing quietly and couldn't bring myself to put my arm around him.

"Court?" he said imploringly. "Put your arm around me."

I just kept crying.

"What is it?" he asked.

I couldn't respond.

He pulled me away from the grave site down a stone path about twenty feet away.

"What is going on?" he asked.

The best answer would've been *Josey died, and I'm sad.* That's the answer a person who hadn't been shoving down her anger for two years and, more important, the past three weeks would've given. That's the answer that a person who could look past her own pain and exhaustion and whatever perceived slight she might have experienced and could recognize that this day was about Josey would've given. I regret to inform you that is not the answer this person gave.

"You should've told me," I said.

"Told you what?" he asked.

"You just should've said, 'Hey, I'm gonna go talk to Kelley for a while. Are you okay? I love you.' You just should've said that."

I watched as all the color, feeling, and love drained from Jake's face. With his head cocked, he squinted at me, looked down, and walked away.

For me, the image of the end of us is simple. It's Jake in a suit, walking wordlessly past a series of gravestones, and me knowing that he would never come back to me.

The heaviness in my chest was almost unbearable, and there was nowhere to find comfort. I was three hours from home, surrounded by Jake and Josey's friends, doing my best to hide my agony. As soon as we got to Josey's parents' house, I grabbed the cordless phone from the kitchen and went to the basement to call my friend Marie.

Trying to communicate was pointless because I was mostly incoherent, but I needed to hear a voice outside of my own head. I've never wanted so much to crawl out of my own skin.

"We're not going to survive this," I said.

"You will, sweetie," she said. "You will."

Good friends know when to lie.

That night, Jake came down to bed wordlessly and turned away from me as we went to sleep. I put my arms around him, but it was like sleeping with a man-shaped two-by-four.

The next morning, he'd already left the room when I woke up. As I lay in bed, I heard him come down the stairs to get something.

"Aren't you going to kiss me good morning?" I asked.

He started back up the stairs, not looking at me. "I'll let you know when breakfast is ready."

I sat in bed, hugging my knees to my chest and staring at the spot on the stairs where he'd been, surprised to discover that it was actually possible for the pain to get worse.

We returned to Portland that day, and for the following week, that was how our communication went. Jake had wanted my help with Josey's Portland memorial, and I arranged the flowers and the photos and created a memorial book, all with a minimum of conversation between us. I was still hosting *Live Wire!* at the time, and the memorial, at a local St. Johns pub, was on a show night for me, so I couldn't stay long.

I knew I'd probably never see Jake again after that night. I approached his friend ND, a photographer who had known him for over a decade, and asked him to take good care of Jake.

"Try to get him to stop smoking," I said through tears. "And get him to lighten up if you can. See if you can get his inner dork to run free."

ND agreed to do what he could and kissed my hand, and I left in tears.

I don't know if things would've been different if I had known how to handle my anger. I spent my life in a houseful of people who were terrified of conflict. I used to watch families scream at one another, then enjoy raucous Thanksgiving meals or mock-punish each other with noogies, but somehow, because that hadn't happened in my house, I never internalized the lesson that you can yell and then have a nice sandwich together when it's all over. I thought if I expressed my anger or frustration to people, they'd stop loving me.

The funny thing is, that became a self-fulfilling prophecy. Not only because I ended up expressing myself at the absolute worst moment imaginable, but also because I didn't do it a million other times at moments that felt small and unimportant but were collectively gigantic.

I couldn't deal with my anger, and Jake couldn't deal with his grief. So it ended.

In a fucking graveyard.

It probably would've ended anyway, years later, when we both hated each other for one reason or another.

But at the time, I was inconsolable. I think it was the one-two punch of losing Josey and the breakup, but for months afterward, I felt like I'd had layers of skin torn off me and I was just wandering around in the world with my organs exposed. If I saw an old man walking an old dog, I cried. If someone cut me off in traffic, I cried. If I got a bad bagel, I cried.

Part of the problem was that, even with everything that had gone down, I still loved him. It's embarrassing and probably quite telling, but I did. I'm sure it had a lot to do with him having been my first... everything. But the fact that I still loved him made it almost impossible for me to accept that we were no longer together. Because movies and songs and poems and books and scrawled messages in beach sand all say the same thing: Love conquers all. I couldn't wrap my brain around the idea that two people could love each other and still be absolutely incompatible in the long run.

Of course I understand that now, but it took me a couple years and a lot of Reese's Peanut Butter Cups to gain some perspective and a lot of the weight I'd lost. When it was all over, I was well on my way to becoming that big girl who didn't want to put herself out there again. Which, at that point, was the safest person to be.

And that's what I became.

Until right before the OFW Project, when I started the whole damn I-think-I'm-finally-ready-to-date thing again.

This time, I hoped, with a little more self-knowledge and a little less self-loathing.

Adventures in Dating I:

Winter, Spring, and How Microsoft Excel Turned Me into an Asshole

Once I'd decided that dating would be a part of the OFW Project, I wanted to use every tool I had at my disposal. I wasn't motivated enough to come up with an algorithm to assess my odds of romantic success, but I assumed the combination of my age and the high percentage of married people in my demographic meant that my dating pool would probably be kiddie-pool-size. I had to throw a wide net, and I had to be fearless about doing so.

Fearless wasn't really my jam, but even so, after kissing off Rich, the guy who wouldn't kiss me, on January 1, on January 4, I posted the following status update on Facebook:

> Friends: I, like millions of people across the country, have recently signed on to a dating site in an attempt not to die alone. If you can help me to avoid going on dates

with strangers who speak about themselves in the third person, please introduce me to your favorite single un-crazy friend (or your single friend who is fucked up in a way that you believe complements the ways in which I am fucked up).

I appreciate your attention to this matter.

You may be thinking, *Wow. How could she possibly post that? I'd be mortified.* Let's look at an equation that explains where I was at the time:

$$L + E[OA] - AG > PTPMLWKDMAL + FDA$$

Or:

Loneliness plus Encroaching Old Age minus the Ability to control Gravity is greater than the Possibility That People in My Life Will Know the Depths of My Aforementioned Loneliness plus Fear of Dying Alone.

I wish there were a different word for the brand of loneliness that comes from being partnerless in a partnered-up world. (*Untethered? Genitally unattended-to? Terminally unaccompanied?*) Some way to quickly communicate the strange juxtaposition of being happily surrounded by people you love and grateful for their presence while periodically sobbing in your driveway after returning home from a party because Gillian Welch's "Dear Someone" grabbed your chest through your car stereo.

It's a loneliness that comes with a tremendous amount of guilt for not recognizing how lucky you are to have the love you *do* have and for behaving eerily like the kind of woman who's so weak that she can't be happy without a man.

I was happy overall. Or at least happy-ish.

I just periodically sobbed in my driveway, and I decided I would rather not do that. That doesn't seem unreasonable. Does it?

So I embarrassed myself on Facebook, and it didn't lead to any set-ups, but it did cause a couple of men who hadn't known I was single to message me. Lesson learned: Increase the number of sly status updates that clue people in to your singlehood, things like *I sure do look silly on this tandem bicycle!* or *I liked* The Revenant, *but I would've enjoyed it so much more if I weren't so desperately lonely.*

I was also on Tinder at that point, which triggered a couple more offers of dates, which also triggered...a thought. And that thought was *How will this not end like the last time? I am bad at this.*

Not *bad* in the sense that I'd been doing it for years and still couldn't catch my snap, just *bad* in the way anyone's bad at something he or she has done just five times. Yes—I really, technically, had been on only about five dates in my life. And now, because of this ridiculous project, I had made a deal with myself that if someone expressed an interest in me and I found him interesting too, I had to agree to a date if he asked me. (I had toyed with the possibility of forcing myself to ask people on dates but quickly ditched that idea because it made me nauseated and no one looks cute while throwing up.)

I wanted to go on as many dates as I could, y'know, for practice, and I needed a good way to document them since my memory had turned to shit in my forties. Also, I had not chosen so well my first time out of the gate, what with the ravaged heart and all, so I needed to figure out a way to look at this next foray more...pragmatically.

So I made a spreadsheet.

I know.

It's truly horrible.

But I honestly believed that if I approached dating with something as cold and scientific as a spreadsheet, I would be more objective, and any resulting relationship would be less likely to fail.

This also meant I could add the ability to freeze header rows to my Microsoft Office skill set. So, win-win?

The categories I created were as follows, each of which were rated on a scale of 1 to 10:

- Smart
- Funny
- Finds Me Funny
- My Attraction to Him
- His Attraction to Me
- Interesting Job He's Passionate About
- Good Conversation
- Sex
- Likes to Talk About Ideas
- My Overall Affection for Him

I realize that this makes me seem, well, dickish. I don't refute that. Rating a person on a scale from 1 to 10? How cold and calculating. I mean, literally calculating. I suppose my only defense[1] is that I believe we all do this in our heads anyway; I just typed it into an algorithm.

I don't expect you to forgive me for this, but I will say that I've adopted three cats and one dog in my life and I once almost gave the

---

1   Massive rationalization.

Heimlich to a stranger in a restaurant but she managed to swallow so it wasn't necessary. What I'm saying is, I'm not all bad.

Plus, I wasn't looking for a perfect score. I just wanted a tool to help me make a choice that wouldn't bite me in the ass later. Or one that would bite me in the ass, but only if I asked it to.

In any case, the spreadsheet was how I moved forward into the strange and not-so-wonderful world of online dating.

I'm now going to outline some of the dates I went on. And I'll include some spreadsheet notes and highlights just to remind you of what a jerk I am.

First Date #1, Early January: Text Guy

Text Guy was someone I'd met through work years before and who had asked me out after reading my humiliating Facebook post. For various reasons, he couldn't meet me in person for a couple of weeks, so we texted each other. Constantly.

He was quick-witted and had a self-deprecating charm that came through even in a medium that's not known for revealing a person's warmth, and I immediately fell deep in like with the digital version of him. So when we finally went out, our corporeal selves had to catch up with how far our text relationship had progressed. I knew all about his family, the years of work he'd invested in his dream of becoming a motorcycle designer, and his most recent heartbreak before I even shook his hand. Oh, and I knew that he was living in his truck.

Well, technically, he was living with his parents after losing his job a few weeks prior, but he didn't like staying there, so he mostly slept in his truck in and around Portland.

Lives in his truck wasn't on my must-have list for a mate, but it didn't really faze me because I liked him so much.

On our first date, he picked me up in his truck (aka house) to take me to sushi and said if things went awry, we could always just turn our backs and text each other.

That wasn't necessary for me. I was even more smitten with him in person.

We had already met years prior, and after the texting, I felt like I knew him, so that helped shrink my dread ball. I had a little bit of buzzing anxiety in the beginning but nothing that threatened to turn into a full-blown anxiety attack.

He was six foot four and athletic with penetrating dark brown eyes, lashes like furry butterfly wings, and a wide, ever-present smile. He was also nine years younger than me. After four dates (one where he spent the whole time trying to warn me off him) and two sleepovers at my place, it became clear he Just Wasn't That Into Me.

But it was confusing. Because if all someone had to go on was our text threads, that person would have thought he was very interested. We spent a good hour or more every day text-flirting back and forth. I think he enjoyed the banter and didn't want to lose that even when he was losing interest physically.

Which he definitely was, but I didn't want to see it because I was so amazed that this handsome, fit, younger guy was paying attention to me.

Originally, I'd rated his sexual attraction to me as a 7 but later I'm pretty sure I saw him cringe when I took my shirt off in the dark so I had to downgrade it to a 2. Perhaps due to his youth, he wasn't used to the fact that things aren't as perky when a woman hits forty. I chose to pretend it hadn't happened, because if I were to accept the reality of that experience, I might not ever be able to take my shirt off again. And a person needs to shower.

The biggest takeaway from the 7-down-to-2 situation: Sometimes the dark is not as dark as you think it is, so be careful what you do with your face. And body. And heart.

After about three weeks, Text Guy ended the relationship via text, which I was initially angry about but in retrospect decided made perfect sense. Our physical selves barely knew each other, while our digital selves were quite intimate, so they were the ones who required a breakup. It was logical, but my physical self was stung.

I'd already had my first minor heartbreak, and it was only January.

Text Guy epilogue: He wanted to remain friends, so we did, because that's what I thought adults did.

We went out to sushi as friends three or four times, and the first two times were miserable for me. Hanging out with friends is supposed to be fun. Sitting across the table from someone you are extremely attracted to but can't fuck is not fun.

On our third sushi friend-date, he showed up having grown a beard that served only to make him significantly more handsome to me. This may be because I've lived in Portland for twenty years, during which time my mental male archetype has grown a beard. (It's a beardy town.)

In any case, now I was even more miserable because I was more attracted to him.

I told myself that I would say no the next time he asked me to go out.

And then he asked me to go out again.

And I said yes. (Don't judge.)

And something magical happened.

This time, he had grown his beard so long that it had a sort of Grizzly Adams vibe. A vibe that I was totally not vibing with. Like, *at all.*

So I sat there across the table from him and listened to him talk, and for the first time, I really heard him.

He talked so much about motorcycles. So much. Why hadn't I noticed this before? And he wasn't the least bit interested in the things I wanted to talk about, changing the subject every time I brought up my work or an article I'd just read.

And that's when I learned what a shallow douchebag I am.

Somehow I had convinced myself that Text Guy and I were totally compatible and that a relationship between the two of us was feasible. I had created a verbal Instagram filter, whereby everything he said got prettied up by his hot, hot face.

In retrospect, Text Guy was a good person to start my dating experiment with because he rejected the shit out of me, and while I had an unpleasant couple of days at the end of January, I didn't immediately die of mortification from liking someone more than he liked me. Getting rejected right out of the gate doesn't feel like an ideal situation, but when one of your goals is to quell your fear of rejection, it kind of is.

High Score: My Attraction to Him

Low Score: His Attraction to Me

Lesson Learned: I am hella shallow and it's totally okay if someone I shouldn't have been interested in in the first place isn't interested in me.

First Date #3, Mid-January: The Ethical Slut

I met the Ethical Slut on Tinder. Of course.

For the uninitiated, Tinder was supposed to be the straight world's answer to Grindr (a hookup app for gay men), but since women were involved, it turned into a dating app but with more hookups per capita than OkCupid or eHarmony.

I wasn't looking for just a hookup, but because I felt so behind, I was hoping to do a cannonball into the dating pool, and Tinder was so ubiquitous at the time that it seemed like it would offer me the most choices.

As a nervous Nellie, what I liked about Tinder was that no one who didn't like me could contact me (both parties must swipe right on, or "like," each other's profiles in order to be able to communicate),[2] meaning I probably wouldn't get horrible, cruel messages telling me to eat some kale or get a neck lift or learn how to handle my finances. Even so, I hovered over the Post Profile button for a good ten minutes before I actually clicked on it.

I spent about a half an hour the first night cringing as I swiped right on profiles, sort of hoping for a match but also sort of not. I got three matches that night, but no messages.

The next day I was swiping right while eating an amazing pulled-pork taco at my desk when I knew I should've been researching an author who was coming on the show to talk about why humans loved

---

2   There are tales of men going through Tinder and swiping right on every profile so they can see who likes them and then decide whom to fuck from that pool. FYI, if you are one of these men, you're a movie villain. Just know that.

water so much. (I might have cared about my job around 15 percent less at this point. But I would never stop caring about pulled-pork tacos.)

I felt a rush of adrenaline when the Ethical Slut messaged me immediately after we matched.

He was an HR rep for a large law firm. He was compact and athletic with a healthy tan, a chiseled chin, and a wild mop of wavy black hair.

He said he wanted to meet me that night.

That felt fast. But I had said I would do this, so I was going to do it, because I said I would do it, did I already say that? My hands felt tingly.

I agreed to meet him after texting eighteen of my friends to ask whether I should meet him.

What if he's a modern Ted Bundy? I texted my friend Allison. *Dating apps seem like an amazing way to find victims.*

No, they're horrible, she replied. *There's a clear digital trail. Have you never watched a police procedural?*

There was still some adrenaline hanging around as I sat at the bar in a Mexican restaurant in Northwest Portland waiting for him. There were chips and salsa in front of me but I didn't want to eat them because my boobs are messy-food magnets. I was grateful that it was the middle of winter and my hands were still cold from walking outside and therefore not clammy. My leg bounced to its own techno drummer. I perused Facebook on my phone and questioned both the OFW Project and dating as a concept.

I took a sip of ice water because eating or drinking, especially eating or drinking something very hot or very cold, can help nervous people focus their attention on their senses and away from their ruminating thoughts. (Ruminating thoughts, in the psychiatric sense, are negative thoughts you should let go of, but can't, like a mental tug-of-war where everyone else at the picnic has moved on and is drinking beer and eating potato salad, and you're still in the mud, holding on to the rope and asking it why you never finished college. They're extremely popular with OCD sufferers.)

The Ethical Slut walked in with purpose and speed, wearing a sharp navy peacoat and a turtleneck sweater. He shook my hand with great vigor and a huge smile on his face. I took a deep breath when I realized he didn't seem at all like a monster.

He sat down and started talking as I took more deep breaths and used my left hand to force my leg to stop bobbing. He clearly had no issues meeting strangers. He was adorable and earnest, and as soon as my mental chatter quieted down and I could actually hear what he was saying, I became fascinated by his no-nonsense approach to dating. He let me know immediately that he was an ethical slut (a term coined in the 1997 book of the same name by Dossie Easton and Catherine Liszt about "consensual non-monogamy") and believed strongly in constant honesty. So constant was his honesty, in fact, that it was jarring.

About twenty minutes in, he leaned into me at the bar, flashed a wide, enthusiastic smile, and said, "I think this is going really well. Do you think it's going well?"

Um. I don't know. There's a lot of stuff going on right now. I'm still trying to figure out what I think of your hair.

"Yeah," I replied. "You seem...nice."

And as much as his ethical-slut thing probably turned a lot of people off, I was being honest. He did seem nice. Really, the nicest slut I'd met in a while.

He told me he'd decided to try consensual nonmonogamy (dating a bunch of people at once and being radically honest about it with all involved) after a conversation with his mother.

"She told me that I'd be really lucky if I found three things," he said. "Someone to socialize with, someone with whom the sex was really good, and a playmate for camping and hiking and stuff."

"That sounds about right," I said.

"Yeah, so I just had a kind of tough breakup from a monogamous relationship, and I'm hoping, ultimately, to find three different women who can each fulfill one of those roles so I won't have to depend on any one of them for everything."

I squinted a little.

"I don't think that's what your mom meant," I said.

He laughed.

"No," I said. "I mean, I really don't think that's what she meant."

"I know," he said. "But it just seems like the safest way to go for me right now."

That made sense to me. Immediately after my one-and-only heartbreak, I would've wanted to keep things light and airy as well if I hadn't waited a fucking decade to date again.

The ES was attractive, and his attitude, charm, and enthusiasm made him a sort of human Labrador, but we didn't necessarily want to talk about the same things. (That night, we talked over nachos about HIPAA requirements regarding e-mail correspondence, which I realize doesn't sound very interesting, but you might be surprised to learn that it's even less interesting than it sounds.)

Still, when he wasn't waxing unpoetic about e-mail legalities, he could be quite entertaining, and the best part was when he made it clear that he was attracted to me, which was refreshing after that yearlong lack of clarity with Rich and then Text Guy's rejection.

After two dates, the ES came home with me and we...enjoyed each other's company greatly. After that, I stopped referring to him as the Ethical Slut and began referring to him as the Cunnilingus Savant.

He was so good at it that I asked him if he would be willing to come to my house and diagram his technique on a whiteboard so I could present it to future dates. He seemed willing, but if I were him, I'd've kept that shit locked up. Dating is competitive, and he had the romantic equivalent of the Coca-Cola recipe. Patent it. Trademark it. Send cease-and-desist orders.

We dated casually for a few weeks, both of us being clear that we were seeing other people and knowing this probably wasn't leading anywhere. In the past, I had only had sex with men I was interested in having a romantic relationship with, and I was surprised at how easy it was, after the initial self-consciousness and apprehension wore off, for me to have an almost purely physical relationship.

In fact, it was kind of a relief that I didn't want a romantic relationship with him. It meant I could just play. Now I understood all those dudes in college who kept sleeping with my friends but had no desire to be monogamous. Emotional attachment is a buzzkill. It gets you all wound up and worried, and the moment you get attached is the moment you start wondering what will ultimately unattach you.

That might just be me.

At one point, he asked me in an e-mail how my other dates were going.

Fine, I suppose, I wrote back. *But I'm so tired. It's exhausting trying to appear charming for this many hours a week.*

I know, he replied. *Dating is exhausting. But if you can find one or two people you enjoy going out with, bringing home, and then sending away so you can get some work done, then that's success.*

I laughed out loud when I read it and responded that that was the most romantic thing anyone had ever said to me.

It was refreshing to see exactly what I didn't want laid out in black and white like that.

It made me think maybe I should let him go and move on, but I didn't really have to because we just sort of faded away from each other.

I was grateful to the Ethically Slutty Cunnilingus Savant, though, for being my very first online date. From then on I was significantly less apprehensive about meeting people because my experience with him had made something crystal clear: Dates were just job interviews with booze and apps. Both people involved have lists of requirements they need fulfilled, and each is just feeling the other out to see if that person has the experience, demeanor, and skill set required.

Of course, dates are (often, but not always) more fun than job interviews, but looking at them that way helped me calm the fuck down, and calming the fuck down and enjoying myself was what the Okay Fine Whatever Project was all about.

High Score: Sex. By a long shot

Complicating Factors: I'm reasonably sure his roommate was in love with him

Lesson Learned: Bring dating CV to bar along with condoms and lube.

First Date #5, Late February: Wait-List Guy

He was a sweet, funny, and curmudgeonly-in-the-most-charming-way advertising creative director who unfortunately started seeing someone exclusively just as we were setting up our first in-person date after chatting on OkCupid. He said he'd meet me anyway, since I was technically grandfathered in.

We met at a bar in my neighborhood and he was, tragically, just as adorable in person as he'd been online: crumpled, world-worn oxford button-down over a T-shirt, scruffy beard, and a baby face that made him look well under his forty-six years. I immediately felt like we had been friends forever, which helped to shrink my dating dread ball to approximately golf-ball size. We talked for three hours that first night, mostly about my dating trials, how much working for corporations sucked balls, and a semi-obscure band we both loved called Slim Cessna's Auto Club.

"We were at a SCAC show together about a decade ago," he said.

"What?" I responded. "We were? Did you just remember that?"

"No," he said. "I was kinda drunk and you were with a friend...a blond woman."

"Marie, yeah," I said, as I remembered standing self-consciously on a makeshift dance floor in a smoke-filled club on Hawthorne Boulevard with a sparse crowd of sweaty, pogo-ing cool kids.

"I told her I thought you were lovely," he said.

"That's insane," I said. "How do you remember that?"

"Well, she told me about *Live Wire!*," he said. "That I should check it out. And I did. So I remember you."

It's always so strange when you have a memory of an event and suddenly you get a whole new piece of information that expands the picture beyond your own experience—like you lived the original script and someone hands you a rewrite. Before, it was just me and my friend geeking out at a tent-revival-like rock show, and now it was a story about missed opportunities.

Now I understood why he'd grandfathered me in—because that's a pretty great story to be able to tell someone you randomly meet on the internet.

In the coming weeks, we drank and chatted a few times. I always kept things totally platonic, but I knew what I was doing was at the very least mildly sketchy.

Why was I hanging out with this man who was already taken? Because I wanted to make sure I was first on the waiting list if that other woman didn't work out. Is that something a sociopath would do? Probably. I was in a dating gray area that was really more bright red and flag-shaped, but our conversation flowed better than on any of my dates so far, and he had *just* started seeing that other woman exclusively a week before we met, so...

Yeah, it still sounds terrible.

Eventually, Wait-List Guy became Sweet Curmudgeonly Friend Guy. He turned out to be a great confidant and very helpful as a primary source for the straight-male-in-his-forties perspective on things. ("Why isn't he texting me back?" "Because he doesn't like you?" "That is brilliant. Thank you.")

He became like a second brother, except that I was once super-attracted to him. So not like a second brother at all. Gross. But a good friend.

High Score: My Overall Affection for Him

Low Score: Myself, as a person, for rating him at all once I really came to like him

Lesson(s) Learned: I might be a sociopath, but sometimes good things can come from the worst intentions.

First Date #8, Late March:
Guy-Who-Doesn't-Know-What-He-Wants Guy

The second of five coders I met on OkCupid, this guy wooed me, immediately disappeared, drunkenly apologized two weeks later, went on a text rant about what assholes people in Portland were (I wasn't sure if I was included or not), asked me out again "as a friend," and then followed me on Twitter when I said, "No, I think I'm good."

Lesson Learned: Maybe stop dating because this is uncomfortable and inconvenient and meeting on the internet is unnatural because you would never otherwise cross paths with these people and isn't it more logical to date humans you actually meet in the real fucking world because that means you have at least one goddamn thing in common that somehow leads you to be in the same physical space?

It was after first date #8 that I deactivated my OkCupid profile for the first time. I knew it was just temporary, but I was tired and just a little demoralized.

Dating was hard. At this point I'd been on twenty-four dates total (I'd been on as many as eight dates with some of these guys), and that felt like plenty for now. Maybe forever.

When I looked over my spreadsheet, I realized that it was flawed for lots of reasons, but one huge one was that I hadn't weighted particular categories more heavily than others.

For me, Good Conversation was far more important than just about any other category, but if someone with whom I'd had a great conversation scored lower in other categories, he would seem, overall, to be a lesser match. If I were better at math or spreadsheets, I could've adjusted for this issue.

I know this is going to sound weird, but I was realizing that maybe rating people on a scale from 1 to 10 wasn't the best idea in the world. Even so, I was still doing it. Something about it gave me comfort, as if an algorithm would be able to solve a mystery that I couldn't crack on my own.

At this point, I wasn't sure I'd ever actually find anyone through online dating, but I was proud of my stick-to-itiveness.

Even so, for a couple of weeks, I was just going to apply that stick-to-itiveness to something else.

Like napping.

A Brazilian in Portland:

Wherein I Discover a Border I'd Rather Not Cross Again

Hair is weird.

Hair on your head makes sense; if you have any bald friends, they can tell you how bone-chilling it is when their shiny pates go uncovered on a cold winter night.

But pubic hair? What possible purpose could pubic hair serve at this point in human evolution?

Theories vary.

Some believe it's a guard against friction in an area subject to skin-on-skin action during the course of the day (or week, or month, or, in the sad case of me in my twenties, never).

According to some sources, it could be a sort of nest for pheromones released by sweat glands that, combined with sebaceous secretions, create what you might call the body's own musky "come-hither."

Still others regard pubic hair on women as the "eyelashes of the vagina," keeping dirt and other detritus from entering their lady-bits.[1] I've never had any stray items fly into my vagina and I've always kept it pretty au naturel, so maybe there's something to this theory.

Regardless of the reason why the hair's there, people can't seem to decide how they feel about it.

I'd thought that the trend of yanking it all out was a new(ish) thing, but shaving and depilatory practices go back to at least ancient Greece, when women would pluck, pumice, and even burn the hair off their nethers with smoldering ash or heated lamps. (I always think that putting a razor near my clitoris is playing with fire, but smoldering ash? That's leveling up.)

King George IV (1762–1830) commingled his lovers' hair in a snuffbox, now kept in a collection at the University of St. Andrews that I assume is titled Gross Shit from History. But he wasn't an outlier. Apparently, nineteenth-century British women used to give pubic hair to their lovers as a fond remembrance.

Right now in America, people are a lot less sentimental about their pubic hair. Mostly, they just want it gone.

Pubic crazes run the gamut from the full-on porn-star/creepy-prepubescent look to the oxymoronic full-bush Brazilian, which means that you take all the hair off the labia but leave what some refer to as "the magic triangle" intact.

In Korea, apparently, a shaved or waxed vagina is not considered

---

1   If by *detritus*, they mean "men who require their girlfriends to get their vaginas waxed before they have sex with them," they may be right. Well done, pubic hair!

attractive. There, pubic hair on women is viewed by many as a sign of health and fertility, so there are women paying up to two thousand dollars to have pubic-hair-transplant surgery, like a vaginal Hair Club for Women.

Don't they know that a decent merkin runs only, like, twenty bucks?[2]

I'd never felt particularly strongly about pubic hair one way or the other, which was evidenced by my lackadaisical approach to my own. I have friends who keep their hedges neatly trimmed regardless of whether they'll have an audience or not, but I am not in that camp. If my hedges were being viewed by someone other than myself, I'd give them a little bit of attention. Otherwise, hey—you do you, labia.

But back in February after my infamous Facebook post inviting all comers, I was embarking on what I hoped would be a robust series of dates that ideally would lead to sexual encounters if all went well, so I figured those areas that had previously been dark and overgrown with the vulval vines of singlehood would need some attention.

At that point I still wasn't the size that I wanted to be, but even after gaining a little weight back, I was still about fifty-five pounds down from my heaviest and feeling confident. Not, like, normal-size-

---

2   A merkin is a pubic wig, worn a few centuries ago by people who had to shave their pubic areas to combat lice or by prostitutes to hide the evidence of an STD. Now they're worn by actors in films so they appear nude when in actuality their nethers are covered. This is largely because full-frontal nudity sends their pay through the roof, and also because actors live for exposure, just not that much.

person confident,[3] but confident. Although that confidence would not necessarily translate to the bedroom, even if my vulva was properly attended to by a waxing professional.

I have always felt self-conscious about my body in the bedroom. So much so, in fact, that it's a miracle that I can enjoy sex at all.

I've got friends who talk about totally losing themselves during the act, but that has never happened to me. I'm still absolutely, 100 percent in my brain no matter what's going on in my vagina.

Whoever I'm with has to be immensely talented to get past my internal monologue.

Don't get me wrong—I enjoy sex, and I can get pretty damned heated. It's just that underneath the heat, there's a bunch of chatter. And 98 percent of it has to do with my body.

It's hard to explain, but this may help illustrate.

A Sample Inner Monologue I Generally Have During the Act of Sexual Intercourse

Mmm . . . this is nice. This is so nice. Jesus, he's a good kisser. What'd I have for lunch today? I should've brushed my teeth before this . . . oh, mmm . . . the neck thing. Nice.

Oh God . . . don't touch the backs of the thighs . . . so gross. [Turns slightly to the side to make cellulite less noticeable.] *That should do it.*

---

3   Before the entire internet comes at me: I realize fat women are normal. But I've been fat my entire adult life, and regardless of how many self-help books I read or how many feminist affirmations I memorize, I will never feel normal, because "normal" is portrayed in the media as a size I will never come close to. And I could stop consuming media in protest, but then what would I do to avoid writing?

Now my stomach looks bad. I'll go back to position one and just deal with the shitty thighs.

I could straddle him, maybe? But then I'll have eight chins when I look down, and my belly will look doughy and I'll have to hold my boobs up.

I could maybe give him a blow job and avoid the whole...oh, okay...he's on my boobs now. The boobs have never done that much for me sexually, but it's nice, I guess. Okay, he's spending some serious time on the boobs. Should I say something? I won't say anything. That'd break the mood. But what if this works out between us? It's not like ten years down the road I can say, "Oh, by the way, my boobs have never really been a big erogenous zone for me. I don't know if it's a surface-area problem or what; I mean, it's pleasant, but it's not, like, earth-shattering." And then he'd say, "I spent a lot of time on your boobs. Now I can never get that boob time back!" And I'd say, "Oh yeah, well, give me all that ball time back! At least boobs are pleasant to be around, but balls? Disgusting!" And he'd say, "Oh, now you're attacking my balls! I knew this would get personal!" And I'd say, "I'm not attacking your balls, I'm attacking balls in general, which I think we can agree are not attractive!" And he'd say, "But I shaved them for you!" And I'd say, "Yeah, doesn't really help. Ever see one of those hair-less dogs? Those things are not cute." And he'd say, "You're comparing my balls to a hairless dog?" And I'd say, "Look, I don't want to have this argument with you... in my head... while we're having sex... ten years ago." Wait... why am I imagining a fight we're going to have in ten years? Oh, because he's been on my boobs for the past five minutes. Right. Okay. I have to distract him.

Blow job!

And it goes on from there.

So you can imagine that if there was anything I could do to increase my odds of not getting distracted by self-conscious brain chatter during sex, I would do it.

Which is why a Brazilian seemed like the perfect addition to the Okay Fine Whatever Project. Maybe it'd give me a bit more self-confidence. A little... vaginal flair, so to speak.

I'd never had one before, largely because of the aforementioned years of singlehood. Well, that and the fact that I have a low threshold for pain and don't enjoy strangers having unfettered access to my hoo-ha. (I'm not ashamed of my vagina; it's perfectly average, I think, based on a reasonably small sample size. It's just that it's one of a couple of private areas on my body where private things happen privately.)

But this was the Year of Doing Uncomfortable Shit™ and maybe if I had the most perfectly coiffed vagina in the world, it would help boost my confidence and quiet my brain a little. So I made an appointment with a place called Wax On Spa, partly because it was specifically recommended for its Brazilians and partly because I dug the *Karate Kid* reference and thought that a sense of humor might be a great thing for your bikini waxer to have.

In case you're unfamiliar with it, a Brazilian is where you have all the hair waxed off your pubic area, including your perineum and everything behind it, leaving only a tiny "landing strip" of hair right in the middle of your pudenda.

Yep. That's what I signed up for.

I walked into the bright, industrial space at Wax On and was simultaneously put at ease *and* terrified by the snifter of tequila on the table in front of me. It managed to signal both *Hey, we're fun and casual about this!* and *This is going hurt like a motherfucker.*

Then I met Laurie, an affable young redhead who has been doing Brazilians for over a decade. Laurie had spent much of her career in Vegas, which I would imagine is the Brazilian capital of the world.

Laurie led me to my own private waxing area, and on the way I passed a room with one of those Obama Hope posters on the wall. I was glad I wasn't in that room, since the experience would've been even more surreal with the president looking aspirationally between my legs.[4]

The poster seemed a little out of place, but when you think about it, getting a Brazilian is a hopeful act for many, like keeping your house clean just in case friends drop by unexpectedly.

Laurie had me undress completely below the belt and gave me the tiniest towel ever made to cover up with, which was kinda funny considering what her vantage point was about to be, but I'm sure she did a lot of things just to help people manage the humiliation. If it makes a person feel better to have her vagina covered by a washcloth prior to someone sticking her face five inches from it, so be it.

She explained to me that she was going to use a wooden tongue-depressor-like tool to spread wax on me, then she would press small strips of fabric onto the wax and rip out all my hair from the roots.

Which I agreed to.

Which begs the question, Why do I hate my vagina so much?

I kid. I don't hate my vagina. But I sure do have a weird way of showing it how much I love it.

---

4   This was prior to the 2016 election, which I don't really want to go into here except to say "Gross."

Laurie was really honest about the pain—she said that of course she couldn't tell me that it wouldn't hurt, but she said the pain was manageable, which it was, largely. Until the very end.

I'm not sure how other Brazilian artists do it, but Laurie worked from the outside in, which I'm sure she did to ease people into the experience, but for me that meant going from the least amount of pain to the most.

I won't get too graphic, but the clitoral hood sort of has its own hood, and there's actually hair on the inside of that. *I would have her skip that next time.* I'd have her skip the whole middle area, really, because the pain got so much worse the closer she got to…central booking. It was like the difference between getting your eyebrows plucked and being impaled on an iron fence.

But that's just me. I'm a person who doesn't want my beauty regime to cause me more pain than a standard dental cleaning.

Laurie said it always hurts the most the first time. (There's another experience involving the vagina that this is true of as well…what is it again?) After that, the hairs become finer and therefore less stubborn. Plus I'd imagine that after the first time, a woman knows what she's in for, so she takes twelve whiskey shots or two hydrocodone or sits on a giant ice block to prepare. Now that I think about it, I have seen a resurgence in old-timey icehouses. I thought it was just another Portland hipster thing, but now I get it.

The experience is made even stranger when you have the same casual chitchat you'd have with your hairstylist or manicurist with someone who's staring at a part of your body even you feel uncomfortable looking at.

It's like when your gynecologist asks you what you did last weekend while she performs a pap smear. It's just not a position that's conducive to opening up. Ironically.

As far as the result, as much as I hate to admit it, it felt pretty great. The skin on your labia is incredibly soft, and with the right pair of silky underwear rubbing up against your business, you can feel borderline Paltrowian.[5]

So I almost understand why women do it. Almost.

I aspire to brain-chatter-free sex, I really do. But in practice, the amount of sexual confidence I gained from my new vaginal haircut couldn't nearly make up for thirty-plus years of constantly comparing myself to an unrealistic feminine ideal and saying horrible things to myself for not meeting it. Not that I thought it would.

If someone invented a pill that would keep women from thinking about what their bodies looked like during sex, they would make more money for the sexual-industrial complex than Hugh Hefner did in his entire career. In a day.[6]

Ultimately, I know it's not really about needing a pill. It's about recognizing that the person you're with is obviously attracted to you in some way or he or she wouldn't be on top of you. Or beside you. Or behind you, or wherever you enjoy having your business worked on.[7] So let go and let

---

5 . Is there a celebrity who feels as amazing as Gwyneth does about her vagina? I don't think so.

6 Booze does this to a degree but it's not effective enough, and too much of it leads to a very sticky nonconsent issue that we won't get into here because it's not well suited to the fun romp of a reading experience my publisher hopes you are having.

7 Yes, sometimes people sleep with you when they're not really attracted to you, but if that's happening on a regular basis, you have bigger problems than body issues and should seek help. For realsies.

Gordon or Jim or Jenny or whoever it is do what he or she does. And you do what you do, without worrying about what your belly looks like while you're doing it. Because no one else is. I can almost guarantee it.

This is all to say, I suppose, that I'm not getting another Brazilian.

Mostly because of all the reasons I've outlined here, but also because, after all of this, it struck me that my choices about the amount of hair I subtract from or add to my pubic area actually affects the person I'm dating more than it affects me. I mean, my face will never be down there unless I get much better at yoga. So if I end up dating a person who's just wildly turned on by vaginas with little sideways Hitler mustaches, then I'll consider it. Otherwise, probably not.

So I learned where I stand on bikini-area grooming, and it led me to pen the following, which I hope will change the world of pubic-hair care for the better. Please pass it along to your sisters.

An Open Letter to Women
Getting Brazilians
And Ruining It for the Rest of Us

Hey, ladies.

Listen, I get it.

There's a lot of pressure out there to appear attractive, so I understand the desire to pluck things and shellac things and even use a wand to apply coats of paraffin, methyl cellulose, and pigmentation to the hair around your eyeballs to make it appear thicker and longer.

No, it's not your fault that our culture has decided that

women's eyeballs don't have enough hair around them and other parts have too much hair, but even so, I think you've gone too far on this one.

I understand that it's complicated down there, and that, in an ideal world, we should make it as simple as possible for others to navigate what can be a dark and confusing place.

But in the same way we currently regret previous generations' razing the rain forests, the women of the future will regret today's women's personal rain-forest razing—seeing it as an era when we could've saved ourselves a lot of pain but chose not to.

Maybe you feel like we're already galloping down the waxing road and it's too late to turn back. Not true. Our culture's hair decisions are clearly arbitrary and reversible. We've moved on from Burt Reynolds's mustache and the dark days of 1980s claw bangs, but we've also gone back and reembraced the mutton-chop and the pixie cut. That means we can go back to a simpler, more accepting time when Afros were all the rage. *Everywhere.*

This is about creating a new cultural contract, one that says: *We all want to be attractive, but we also agree that our personal-hygiene rituals should never trigger a fight-or-flight response.*

Women can do this if we band together. All we have to do is decide, as a gender, that pain hurts and we will no longer pay seventy dollars to have another woman tell us about her boyfriend's weird mole while ripping hair out of a spot we don't even allow ourselves to look at because, frankly, it resembles the alien from *Alien,* and nature has provided natural cover for it, which we should use. And men can make the same contract with other men about hair on their backs and chests and balls (which we've already established are also alien-y), and we can become a culture of happy, furry people, indistinguishable from our prehistoric ancestors aside from the cell phones and rampant narcissism.

We will go back to our roots, which we will also stop dyeing! Eventually.

When I'm ready.

And we'll be content. Until we find something else to feel terrible about. Which will be really, really soon.

Thank you.

Adventures in Dating II:

Summer, the Season of Underboob and Back-of-Knee Sweat

I reactivated my OkCupid profile in May and had a few decent encounters that helped usher me back into the dating world.

There was an insanely smart truck driver who bought me a really delicious cheese plate and somehow made traveling around the country alone sound appealing. There was a guy who worked for public radio that I was excited to meet because we obviously had some shared interests, but I learned as he talked (and talked and talked) that common interests do not equal compatibility. And then there was the sex addict who I didn't end up sleeping with because engaging in co-dependent behavior on first meeting someone seems ill-advised.

What follows are just a few other highlights of summer.

First Date #11, Early May: Outdoorsy Guy

While you're thinking what a jerk I am for putting men into a spreadsheet, it may comfort you to know that once I hit May, the guy with the highest score so far ended up giving me the comeuppance I deserved, largely because I'd left off possibly the most important category of all: Totally and Completely Not into Me.

I only went on a single date with him, but I found him incredibly intriguing. He was laidback, attractive in a burly "Chris Pratt circa early *Parks and Rec*" kind of way, and disarmingly easy to talk to.

His job was to climb the tallest trees in Oregon and measure them. I couldn't believe that was even a job, which is why he became my first 10 in the Interesting Job category.

He was available only during the day on a Saturday, which in retrospect was a clear indication that he wasn't that interested. People who date a lot usually reserve their prime dating times (evenings, especially weekend evenings) for top-tier prospects. But I failed to spot the red flag.

We met at an ice cream parlor, which is a little problematic on a date due to the whole licking-while-talking issue, but we dealt with it.

We talked about how sexy we both found Tina Fey and about how he got into his line of work, and he told me that tree lovers are hiding the world's tallest trees from the public.

"What do you mean, hiding them?" I asked.

"Well, they've found them, but they're not going to tell anyone where they are."

"Why not?"

"Because people are dicks?" he said.

"That's accurate," I said. "But seriously."

"No, seriously," he said. "The tallest tree in the world is somewhere in Redwood National Park—it's three hundred and seventy-nine feet tall and nicknamed Hyperion, but because people can't resist turning trees into tourist traps and then possibly killing them, they'll never reveal where it is. There are more trees like this than you might imagine."

My favorite dates were where I both enjoyed myself and learned a fun fact to use at cocktail parties, so I considered our date a raging success.

He texted me after the date to thank me for being "funny and cool." I told him it was no problem.

We bantered over texts for a week or so—with me initiating most of the time—but he never mentioned wanting to see me again, and then he was just gone.

When I look back on it, I can't believe I thought we were compatible. Yes, talking to him was a pleasure, but almost every one of his profile pictures was of him somewhere high up, near a tree or in a tree or—my personal favorite—dangling on a hammock attached with carabiners to the side of a cliff.

This guy engaged in my worst nightmare for fun, but because I'd had a lovely time chatting with him, I somehow concluded we should date. It was the same situation as the verbal Instagram filter I'd used with Text Guy; it's just that in the case of Outdoorsy Guy, I was blinded to the wild incompatibility of our daily lives by our conviviality and his ability to offer me NPR-quality cocktail-party fodder.

It was just one date, but I was definitely disappointed when he ghosted me.[1] Turns out, I didn't need more than one date for it to sting when I found out that I rated lower on someone's figurative spreadsheet than he did on my literal one.

Lessons Learned: REI has a co-op membership program; tree people have to hide trees to keep the public from turning them into garbage-laden World's Largest Ball of Yarn–style roadside attractions; and I should not date people whose favorite thing to do makes me dizzy when I think about it.

First Date #14, Early July: White-Linen-Suit Guy

I met White-Linen-Suit Guy at a sweet little hole-in-the-wall taqueria in the Alberta Arts District.

He was an artist and a stockbroker, which I thought was an unusual combination, but that's only because I use the fact that I'm a right-brain type to excuse my own financial ineptitude.

All I knew about him before we met was the stockbroker part, which made the white-linen suit a little jarring. (I guess I was expecting pinstripes, not something out of a Tennessee Williams play.) He was about five foot ten, quite tan for someone living in Portland, and had the authentic smile and easygoing affect of a real live hippie. He was also wearing a fedora.

I had no idea what to do with that last piece of information.

---

1   If you've never been ghosted, it's when there's no real end to a coupling; one or both people simply disappear from text communication. Sometimes there's an "illness" or "business trip" involved. I've been ghosted a few times, and I'm embarrassed to say I've been the ghost as well (strep throat, Detroit).

Strangely, at this point in the game I was getting more nervous at the outset of dates instead of less. Once I'd started to think of dates as job interviews, I'd begun to relax considerably, but around first date #12, I noticed that I was getting a bit of dry-mouth and my palms were sweating. I attributed the latter to the fact that it was summer, but it was definitely a thing to worry about (and I was always on the lookout for those).

My palms were sweating with White-Linen-Suit Guy, but thankfully, hand-holding would be far more freaky on a first date than fucking, so I was in the clear.

I hadn't been that excited to meet WLSG because I thought I wouldn't have a lot to talk about with a stockbroker, but he'd made me laugh over messenger on OkCupid, so I thought I'd give him a chance.

I'd been frustrated of late by the fact that, aside from Outdoorsy Guy, it had been more and more difficult to find someone I was conversationally compatible with. But it shouldn't have surprised me that a person who'd spent the past eleven years writing comedy for a radio variety show might have trouble finding conversational common ground with someone who wrote computer code or managed a medical office or just generally existed in the real world with normal people who have to work for a living.

I found myself saying things like "Oh. You have to be at work on time? Every day? What's that like?" or "What do you mean you've never filed an expense report for otter costumes?"

So I settled in at the taqueria for a couple hours of polite nodding, but there was almost none.

White-Linen-Suit Guy was quite funny in person, and about

twenty minutes into the date, he asked me if I'd ever tried ayahuasca.

There are a couple things that might happen when you hear this question. One, the person might be about to ask you if you'd like to join him in an ayahuasca ceremony. This will involve a shaman and will take anywhere from four to eight hours to complete. And you will probably vomit. Or, two, a person is about to tell you about his latest ayahuasca journey, which also might take anywhere from four to eight hours.

In my case, it was the latter.

Since I'd never heard of ayahuasca, it was actually quite interesting. But it did drag on.

If you've never heard of it, ayahuasca is a psychotropic, plant-based brew that has traditionally been used by indigenous Amazonian people as spiritual medicine and shamanic communication but has recently been called "the Drug of Choice for the Age of Kale" by *The New Yorker.*

WLSG described the beginning of the ceremony with the shaman and his own skepticism and then illness after drinking the brew.

"Most people throw up," he said. "I threw up about eight times over the course of a couple hours."

"That sounds horrible," I said.

"It was," he said. "But I'd do it again in a second."

"Why?" I asked.

He went on to describe an experience wherein he found himself on a previously unknown plane of existence, one on which he was able to clearly see his entire life and the people in it, including his daughter and his ex, with whom he'd been embroiled in a nasty divorce.

"In the beginning," he said, "I was watching all the best moments from our lives together like really good TV."

"Nice," I said. "You got to binge-watch your life."

"Yeah," he said. "And then I suddenly felt about her like I used to feel. And I could see the pain she was in now, and my bad feelings toward her just...ended."

"Even when you came out of it?" I asked.

"Yeah," he said. "Right now, I still feel the same way."

"So you can still see things exactly as you did on the drug?" I asked.

"Totally."

I've never been great with drugs (you can imagine why), but if there were a drug that didn't force me to hang out with some dude named Aspen who called himself a shaman, didn't make me vomit for hours, and allowed me to forgive everyone who's ever wronged me, I'd take it in a second. Because I don't want to continue to hold a grudge against that woman who didn't give me "the wave" after I allowed her to merge in front of me on I-5 in 1997; it's just in my nature.

White-Linen-Suit Guy and I walked on Alberta Street for a few blocks after we had drinks and I kept thinking about the idea of being magically brought back to a time when you loved someone you'd later come to hate. Was the experience unnatural or natural? Was the drug manipulating the space-time continuum to erase every moment that ever changed your feelings? Or was it somehow returning you to the kindest, most forgiving version of yourself?

We sat on a park bench for a while talking about the huge market for a forgiveness drug. (I said we could call it Absolvet and use "Let It Go" from *Frozen* as the jingle.)

I knew I'd probably never see him again because we were very different and, I think, only mildly interested in each other, each of us regarding the other as the human equivalent of a plain doughnut: a nice treat if it's the only thing left in the box, but, y'know, fuck plain doughnuts otherwise.

Even with that in mind, I still had an altogether pleasant and illuminating evening, one that the snark machine inside my brain never would've predicted. If this dating binge was doing anything, it was slowly chipping away at the part of me that assumed the worst about people. I now saw that this habit was partly a product of my anxiety, which kept me constantly bracing for the next crisis, and partly a cop-out, because it was easier than actually trying to figure out who people were.

As exhausting as it was, dating was teaching me to be slightly less of an asshole. And I appreciated that.

Then, when I got home from my date with WLSG, I opened my spreadsheet and entered his scores, and suddenly I was an asshole again.

It was a roller coaster of a night.

High Score (if the Category Had Existed): Storytelling

Lesson Learned: Stockbrokers aren't all buttoned-up types—some go on really vomit-y emotional vision quests, and there are some men who can wear the shit out of a fedora.

First Date #18, Late July: DJ Jazzy Jazz Guy

Remember those sweaty palms I'd noticed at the beginning of the month? Later on in July, I developed another new nervous tic. It hadn't ever happened to me before, but after my date with DJ Jazzy Jazz Guy, it seemed destined to become my body's go-to method for making an unforgettable first impression.

It was a reasonably hot day in late July, and we were sitting outside in the crowded, tiki-bar-esque atmosphere of the back patio at a bar called the Bye and Bye. Sunny, and perhaps in the mid-eighties, but not really hot enough to sweat in the shade. For most people.

At the beginning of the date, I'd felt the chest buzzing and shakiness in my arms and hands that were often precursors to a full-blown anxiety attack. But what would be the reason for it? I'd been dating for seven months now; my body and brain had had more than enough time to get used to it. The only explanation I could come up with was that all of this new activity over the course of those months had triggered my GAD to show up inappropriately. (That's one of the many fun things about GAD—sometimes it barges in during experiences that have never caused you concern before and never will again. It's like your nervous system is throwing a twenty-sided die with life events on it to decide when to get agitated.)

I recognized the symptoms, but the mild electrical current on the surface of my skin and the chest tightness both felt like they were holding pretty steady, so I just breathed, drank my vodka and soda, and tried to keep everything at its current level—sometimes "no escalation" was the best I could hope for.

The good news is that the anxiety attack never came.

But sweat did. A lot of it.

I was wearing a low-cut sundress with spaghetti straps, and when the sweating started, I could feel it running down the sides of my head almost immediately. It felt like I was in the shower.

Once the rivers of sweat gushed down from the top of my head, they formed two tributaries, one below each ear, and flowed into a giant estuary that ran down the middle of my cleavage to a great salt lake beneath the center of my bra.

DJ Jazzy Jazz Guy was a sweetheart, a bald and bearded former jazz DJ and current podcaster who wore rockabilly shirts and a wide grin. I was trying to enjoy talking to him about the glory days of radio, but I was too busy ruminating about my flop sweat. How bad was it? Was my hair color turning the rivers red? Did he think I was dying?

I tried to figure out what sort of subtle gestures I could make with my hands to cover the surface runoff coming from what felt like every pore.

"So how many years were you a DJ?" I asked.

"About a decade," he said.

Normal me would've recognized that we had a commonality there, but flop-sweat me was preoccupied with figuring out how I might cover or dry or otherwise obfuscate this thing that I knew was utterly un-obfuscate-able.

I could use my arm to cover my cleavage, but then he could still see my neck, and if I used my other arm to cover my neck, I would look like a hip-hop artist triumphantly crossing her arms after a successful dance battle.

My hairline was totally soaked now, and I knew there were beads of sweat dangling off it. I felt sweat running all the way down my back and into my ass crack. At this point, I became concerned about drowning.

Then, without warning, it just stopped. Like a faucet had been turned off.

But it didn't matter. The damage had been done.

I honestly don't remember anything of significance from that conversation because I was totally engrossed in Flop Sweat Gate '15 for most of it.

Finally, the evening cooled down and I dried off a little and managed to relax. I thought, *Well, he either likes sweaters or he doesn't.*

Turned out, he liked sweaters.

Shockingly, after that inauspicious beginning, DJ Jazzy Jazz Guy and I spent a lovely month drinking summery cocktails and enthusiastically making out. Then I had to take a break to focus on my work, and we just fizzled out.

But I'll always be grateful to him for seeing past my tidal wave of humiliation.

After that experience, I thought I could survive just about anything on a date.

That theory would be tested later on, but in the meantime, I recorded stats for First Date #18.

High Score (in a Category I Created for Him): Ability to Ignore Another Person's Patently Obvious Uncontrollable Physical Event.

Lessons Learned: If you sweat enough on a hot afternoon, once the sun goes down you can actually freeze from sitting in a wet dress, which is why you should always bring a jacket. Also, it turns out you can have a pretty gigantic anxiety event on a date and things can still work out as long as you're with a sweetly forgiving person.

At this point in the OFW date-a-thon, I was definitely disappointed with how things were going. Not only had I not found it—the spark or connection I was looking for—I hadn't found anything even in that neighborhood. But we all know that dating is just a series of horrifying disappointments right up until it isn't.

I was frustrated, but I wasn't ready to quit. Even though some people around me thought it was probably time to.

One afternoon in early August I was sitting in my backyard with a group of friends chatting over drinks, and one of them asked what was going on with me.

I imparted a few of my dating escapades from the weeks prior—using the ridiculous monikers I'd given all my OkCupid paramours, like Weirdly-Obsessed-with-Sake Guy or Pretty-Sure-He-Hates-Me Guy.

She listened for a while, then said, "Okay, well, do you have any stories that don't revolve around looking for a man? Like, stories about other stuff you're doing with your life?"

Her message was clear. She thought I was better than this.

But I wasn't. I'm not.

I'd spent most of my life un-entangled in an entangled world, and I could tell by the way she talked to me that she had no idea what that was like.

I actually liked being alone. I'd been alone twenty-three of my twenty-five adult years, so it was something I knew how to do. I was good at it—probably way better than she was. (I know being alone isn't a competition, but if it were, I would totally win.)

Unless you've been on your own for as long as I have, you don't know what it's like to watch movies and read books and listen to music constantly barraging you with the message that romantic love should be every human's ultimate life goal and if you don't have it, there is something broken about you and maybe you should consider not leaving the house because you're just making everyone sad. Unless... are you seeing anyone right now? Have you met someone? Have you tried to meet someone? You should really try to find someone. Or just stop looking because that's when they'll show up. It'll happen. Or it won't. You should make it happen. Look, but also don't look is what we're saying. Like, try to make it happen and then back off, but don't totally back off so the universe knows you still want it but not so much that it's pathetic. Because wanting it is really sad but having it is really important so try, but don't try. And maybe lose a little weight. Or a lot.

In a world that values monogamous romantic relationships so much more than it does autonomy, it's impossible not to internalize the message that there's something deeply wrong with you if you've been single for an inordinate amount of time (like the majority of your adult life).

All of this is to say, I understood that my friend wanted me to be a better person, not someone who was so desperate to be in a relationship that she'd spend the majority of her summer weekends attempting to fulfill that goal.

I wished I were better than that too. In fact, I wished the whole world were better than that.

But it wasn't, and I definitely wasn't.

Should I have spent some energy parsing how much I actually wanted to be with someone and how much I just wanted to stop feeling like a freak? Probably. But I frankly didn't have time. I had more dating to do.

That being said, the dating I was doing wasn't working.

Was I going about this all wrong? Should I attempt to game the system in some way?[2] Or should I just stop altogether for a while to recombobulate and strategize? I mean, really, what was the rush? Aside from the fact that in our culture, women became invisible right around their forty-eighth birthdays, so I had two years until I disappeared.

I'd heard friends tell horror stories about being on dating sites for three and four years with no success. There was no possible way I could continue doing this for four years. I'd have to get one of those teeth-whitening cheek retractors to freeze my mouth into a smile.

I decided to stick with it, but I needed a new strategy. I took a little break from dating and put my energy into work. And doing drugs. And doing drugs at work.

---

2 There's a very helpful TED Talk by a woman named Amy Webb who gamed the hell out of the online dating system. She generated a seventy-two-point compatibility matrix, then created ten fake male profiles to study her most successful competitors; she eventually developed the perfect profile to attract the perfect man. She's married now. I don't have that kind of dedication. Except to potatoes. I really like potatoes.

Getting Legally High:

In Which I Learn That Some People Just Shouldn't Smoke Pot

The first time I tried pot, I wound up in the hospital.

The hospital.

Because of *weed.*

I was a junior in high school living in Monterey, California, on the Presidio army base. We lived in a big hundred-year-old box of a house that looked like every other house on our street.

My friend Laura Cohen and I were in the attic room that had been my brother's before he went away to college. We had to go out the back door and climb some creaky-ass stairs to get in—it was a dark, windowless room with mud-brown carpeting and a huge built-in desk with a long counter that we sat cross-legged on, because that's how you sit when you "do weed."

We shared half a joint.

After about twenty minutes, I started feeling tingly and mildly dissociated. I was restless and my parents weren't home, so Laura and I went to the main part of the house so I could try to calm down. Sitting was torture, so I walked from room to room, rubbing and then shaking my arms as if the tingling sensation in my chest and limbs could be jiggled or wrung out. Thoughts looped in my brain uncontrollably.

What if this is permanent? I thought. *What if the pot flipped a switch I won't ever be able to turn off?*

Laura and I ended up calling my friend Mary for help. She and her mother arrived about twenty minutes later and took me to the hospital, where a very annoyed doctor put me in a cavernous, darkened exam room under a blanket so I could calm down.

"Why do people *do* this?" I asked him.

Even in my altered state, I felt like it was important to make it clear to the doctor that this was a new experience for me, that I was a good girl and not a *pot addict.*

"I have no idea," he said, shaking his head, jaw clenched.

He hated me so much. But to be fair, my "weed overdose" was probably keeping him from a guy with a half-inch pipe in his head or a really cool vestigial-tail removal.

Later, Mary's mother called my mother, concerned that I had a drug problem. Mary had told her mom that I'd only smoked pot, but, like any self-respecting person who'd come of age in the sixties, Mary's mother doubted that anyone was such a fucking lightweight that she had to go to the emergency room after smoking a joint. She figured I must've smoked crack or something.

Nope. Just pot.

Looking back, I realize that was probably my first anxiety attack.

The problem with weed is that many of the things it can do to your body (rapid heart rate, dizziness, shallow breathing, dry mouth, paranoia, and dissociation) happen to be the exact same things an anxiety attack does. This is why panic is one of the most commonly reported side effects of weed, right after euphoria and ill-advised Funyun purchases.

I always knew I was "high-strung" as a kid, but I'd never had a full-on anxiety attack until that moment. Of course, I didn't know what an anxiety attack was, so I just chalked it up to Nancy Reagan being right about drugs.

I tried weed again in college and had a similar reaction, which is why I'd steered clear of it for most of my adult life.

Until the OFW Project, when I decided that smoking weed for work would be a good idea.

At that point, it'd been over a year since the OCD episode that prompted my leaving my host job at *Live Wire!* and almost a decade since the one before that. As much as I'm a pessimist, I wanted so badly not to have an anxiety attack that I lived in a perpetual state of denial that I'd ever have another one.

Humans are so strange. The things we forget. The things we tell ourselves.

If animals watch a tiger rip their mom apart, they remember that and know they should probably steer clear of the next tiger they see. But not humans. At least, not if the tiger is fun to hang out with in some way, like, say, heroin is.

Anyway, I decided legal weed belonged in the Okay Fine Whatever Project. And it seemed like a good idea at the time.

I did have a reason. I can't say it was a good one, but it was a reason.

I'd been creatively stuck for a few months. I'd worked for *Live Wire!* for eleven years, and I'd written hundreds of sketches. Nothing felt new anymore. I wasn't compelled to create; I just had to. And not all the joy was gone, just most of it.

The glass was approximately one-eighth full.

And the worst thing about it was that I led a team of writers, so whatever the opposite of inspiring is? I had become that.

I should say that writers' meetings were sometimes quite fun but were more often difficult for me to manage emotionally. When we began the show, there were writers who didn't trust my judgment and made it clear to me immediately. (Someone once wrote in an e-mail during a heated discussion about a rejected sketch that he'd "just have to learn to write things that middle-aged women find funny.")

After that, I always sat in writers' meetings with a chip firmly planted on my shoulder (pad, 'cause I'm a middle-aged lady), making the later writers pay for the lack of faith the first ones had. I often shut down discussions if they disagreed with me because I was still trying to prove my worth to people who were long gone.

It's the thing I regret most about my work on the show.

As I write this, I'm sincerely thinking about what I can send those guys to apologize. Does a fruit bouquet say *Sorry my own internalized misogyny and misdirected resentment quashed your sense of creative freedom for a decade?* Maybe just some gift cards.

I wasn't all strident and shitty; I did have some skills. I was an adept editor of other people's work and had a keen ability to imagine exactly how the pitched sketches would play out in front of our fleece-covered-and-left-leaning audiences, a type that I'd gotten to know quite well over the years.

But I was running out of ideas, and I think my co-workers could see the sad quarter inch of water in my glass, and it felt like I was draining their glasses too.

At the same time, I'd been head writer with Luke as host for a year, which was starting to get difficult, as he'd begun to assert himself more than he had initially.

When he first took over as host, he was happy to simply do whatever we gave him, but as the show wore on, it needed to reflect who he was, not who I was, which made perfect sense. He got involved in the writing process, and the show's material became a little disjointed as everyone tried to bend and twist it around a new voice.

I needed to shake things up.

That's where the weed came in.

It may not have been the smartest idea, but when something you once loved doing becomes dry and rote, you'll do almost anything to get that love back. Plus, I was already in the groove of dipping my toe into weird new pools and sensory-deprivation tanks.

Maybe my brain on drugs would be different this time. Maybe I was slowly learning that everything would be okay.

Maybe.

At the time, each *Live Wire!* show had a theme, and this particular week, the theme was "gonzo." Weed was legal in Washington State, so I got the idea that as a tribute to Hunter S. Thompson's gonzo journalism, our entire writing staff should try to write while stoned.

Because no one ever in the history of comedy has written jokes stoned.

But for real, I figured it probably didn't happen a lot in public radio. Garrison Keillor was still hosting *A Prairie Home Companion*, and I doubted that he and Peter Sagal were sparking up fatties to write "News from Lake Wobegon" or "Not My Job" on *Wait, Wait...Don't Tell Me!*

So that's why we felt at least a little like trailblazers.

Get it? Trail*blazers?*

I'm super-down with the weed lingo.

I traveled with Jason Rouse, a *Live Wire!* writer and friend, all the way to Vancouver, Washington (fifteen minutes from Portland), where we purchased a few strains from an adorable little store called Main Street Marijuana.[1]

The place was packed, with small groups of people being helped by about five weed experts, each of whom was wearing a lanyard with a laminated name tag. It was like an Apple Genius Bar but for sweet Mary Jane.

Reefer. Chronic. Wacky tobacky. Fatty boom blatty. Cat's gym shoes.

I made that last one up.

There were glass cases in the front of the store that held weed-infused edibles like brownies, truffles, and even weed soda (soda pot?), then different strains in cases along the walls with samples laid out so you could see the buds.

The paraphernalia were in the center of the store for impulse buyers to grab. There were some adorable Kate Spade–looking polka-

---

1   Weed is legal in Oregon now, and don't think our entire state wasn't filled with shame that Washington beat us to the marijuana-legalization punch. So humiliating.

dot pipes, which made me think that soon we'd have some celebrity cannabis-accessory lines: Matthew McConaugh–bongs. Or On the Bowl Again pipes by Willie Nelson.

As I considered the marketing possibilities, we made our way to the first available salesperson, a woman in a pink hoodie with bright purple hair who, based on her knowledge of the product, was clearly a longtime weed connoisseur.

One thing I love about pot being legalized is that knowing a lot about weed, something that used to make a person unemployable and even prosecutable, is now a skill one can proudly put on a résumé. I imagine this is a distressing fact for people who work for the state agencies regulating pot who have to interview and hire weed experts.

I see you've been growing hydroponic weed in your garage for the past fifteen years . . . you must really know your stuff! [Smiles nervously, digs her nails into her palms to keep herself from calling the FBI.]

We told Lana, our weed genius (or Wenius™[2]), what we were doing and she recommended a couple of sativas—Blue Dream and Dirty Girl. Sativas supposedly lead to an active, creative high.

I told her I was a pot wuss and had experienced anxiety attacks in the past, and she recommended an indica strain, which was more calming. ("This one totally gets rid of my road rage," said Lana. *How is this something you're casually telling a stranger and where are the police?* said my brain.)

We also picked up an indica/sativa hybrid called Joocy Froot. You know, for science.

As you talk to your Wenius (okay, they're really called budtenders, but

---

2   Wenius isn't really trademarked. Or a thing. At all.

I'd like to offer up Wenius for consideration if *budtender* doesn't stick), she writes your order on a sheet, which is then circulated to another budtender to pick up from the back. Like a shoe store but for drugs.

As we stood in the back of the store waiting for our pot that was totally legal, I looked around and decided that Disneyland was full of shit: *This was the happiest place on Earth.* All the customers, to a person, looked like wide-eyed kids on Christmas morning.

For me? How did you know?

Well, you're wearing a Phish T-shirt and you have Legalize It *tattooed on your neck, so. Yeah.*

Finally, our weed was ready and our budtender asked us if we had any questions.

Talking to him reminded me of going to the pharmacist.

"Have you ever taken Alaskan Thunderfuck before? Side effects include becoming awesome. Also, you should always take it with Totino's Pizza Rolls."[3]

He handed us our bag with a smile and we were off.

It was the strangest experience to walk out of a store with a brown paper bag filled with a previously-illegal-and-still-illegal-fifteen-minutes-away product in beautifully designed little baggies and jars.

To walk in, say, "Good day, fine sir! I would like your finest strain of marijuana, please," and walk out with what I asked for was a far cry from someone whispering, "Smoke?" to me in Washington Square

---

3   He did not say this. He just told us which ones had the highest THC and how much to take to avoid freaking the fuck out. Which I appreciated and needed.

Park at midnight. There's something to be said for good lighting and neither party being arrested.

As we left the store, I noticed the font of the logo on the door.

"Ugh. Who still uses Zapf Chancery?" I asked Jason.

"You need to get high and loosen the fuck up," said my employee.

We got into the car with our booty, never giving a thought as to whether we'd run into the po-po, and drove back to the office, where I filled out an expense report. For *weed*.

That evening, I went home and prepared a hummus and cheese plate for my workmates who were about to come over to get high and try to write.

Thankfully, my housemate, Shelly, was a weed connoisseur, so she had plenty of paraphernalia for us—pipes, rolling papers, a giant ceramic bong that looked like something you'd see in the hands of a bearded gentleman in a hot tub in the seventies.

My fellow writers—Andrew Harris, Sean McGrath, and Jason, all extremely entertaining men in their mid- to late thirties—arrived and we set out to do our "work." These guys were all sketch-comedy writers from way back and their banter always sounded like a Quentin Tarantino film without the splattered brains, so I had high (get it?) hopes.

It didn't go well.

Especially for me.

I started off the night by telling the guys what the plan was: I would write any sketch ideas on a whiteboard I'd brought out, and I would also be transcribing as much of our conversation as I could on my laptop.

Jason, the one who'd driven to the weed store, did the prep work, grinding the buds in a crusher to separate the stems and seeds from the flower, then packing them into the bowl of the pipe, a hollow at the end of the glass with a hole in the bottom. I tell you all of this so that even fellow GAD sufferers, straight-edgers, and/or super-dorks who smartly stay away from drugs know what to picture.

We all took initial hits off our chosen strains and then I tried to initiate a sketch-brainstorming session. These almost never worked at *Live Wire!*, so ours quickly devolved into a weird, pot-infused work party.

You know those anxiety attacks brought on by the fear that you're about to have an anxiety attack? Well, if you don't, they're a thing. They're called anticipatory anxiety attacks and they're dicks. I started having them almost immediately after my first cough-filled exhale.

About thirty minutes in, as the guys were talking about a movie with a machine-gun massacre in it, I went into the kitchen to get more ice. As they described the violent scene, I got a rush of adrenaline that immediately turned into panic. I stood at the counter and worried about the knives in the drawer in front of me. The top of my head tingled. I breathed deeply. I wished they'd stop talking about the fucking movie.

I walked back over to the party and started typing some of the things they were saying. My fingers on the keyboard helped, in the same way drinking water had helped on that first Ethical Slut date. Anything that connected me to the physical world eased the panic. Anxiety can be like an electrified fence between you and reality, so bringing even tiny pieces of sensual reality inside that fence helped. So did eating, writing, wiggling my toes on the carpet. Interacting with other people could also help, so I started writing ideas I heard on the whiteboard and asking questions, even though I couldn't really process the answers. (Anxiety is loud.) The bonus of doing this was that it made me seem like a normal human being on the outside. Or at least I assume it did.

As soon as the first wave of anxiety hit, a wave of regret and sadness joined it.

Why did I do this? Now I'm going to be anxious forever, I thought. *Fuck you, Hunter S. Thompson.*

Every time an attack ends, I somehow make myself believe it was my last. And as soon as a new one starts, I'm positive I will never stop having them.

The first one finally subsided, and I thought I might get lucky and not have another one. I decided immediately that I wouldn't take another hit but that a Xanax and a double vodka would also be a fitting tribute to Hunter.

I had about four more mini-attacks—during which I kept breathing deeply and clawing my way through the layers of adrenaline and intrusive thoughts telling me, for example, that there might someday be a Lifetime Movie based on the night's horrific events called *Deadly Funny: The Courtenay Hameister Story*—before the Xanax kicked in, tempered nicely by the vodka.[4] A few times, the meeting became one of those movie scenes where the world goes silent and slow and the protagonist can see people's mouths moving and watch them throw their heads back in laughter, and it's as if she's watching her own life like a silent film she can't get back into.

---

4   Note: I do *not* recommend this combination and, in general, do not recommend drinking in order to deal with anxiety. Cognitive-behavioral therapy, mindfulness, exercise, and prescribed medications have all proven successful in treating anxiety. I didn't have a lot of these tools at the time, so I chose the "either this will work or I'll end up choking on my own vomit" option. Not smart.

I breathed more. And more deeply.

The only way to come back from an anxiety attack is to calm yourself down, and the whole reason you're having an anxiety attack is that you can't calm down. It's fucking torture.

But thanks to chemistry and the discovery of fermentation, the torture finally ended after about an hour.

My co-workers remained unaware that anything unusual or unpleasant was happening to me. It's completely bizarre that what registers as such an earth-shattering event internally can be almost entirely undetectable externally. This is probably one of the reasons mental illnesses are so misunderstood and why people who have them are often not believed or have to prove they're sick to family members who claim it's all in their heads. (This is what my grandfather said about my father's bipolar disorder, and fighting this assertion was difficult because he was technically right about where my father's disease was located.) In one way, a physical manifestation would be nice so people would be more likely to see anxiety as a "real illness," but I'm glad sufferers can make it invisible some of the time. Comes in pretty handy.

As I gradually rejoined reality and registered what I was typing, it became clear that this wasn't the most successful experiment we'd ever run.

I still have my notes from the evening.

Here's what I was able to capture:

7:50: Jason and Sean both try sativas. I ask how many "tokes" it takes to get stoned and get laughed at. I try an indica due to anxiety, and Andrew tries a hybrid.

8:10: Conversational snippet:

> **JASON:** I don't trust him. He wrote me a note in highlighter.
>
> **SEAN:** Writing notes in highlighter is like a serial killer move. It's like having no eyebrows.

8:50: I have my first mini-anxiety attack and we come up with a theme for our next show: Outsiders and Outcasts. That sends us down a rabbit hole about a remake of *The Outsiders* starring hip-hop duo Outkast and wondering whether André 3000 would play Sodapop or Pony Boy.

9:30: No sketch ideas yet. Sean asks me to call for pizza. I make Sean call because talking to strangers on the phone makes me feel weird.

9:32: Business idea: A service you call that will call and order stuff for you.

> **JASON:** Need to order something, but feel weird?
>
> **ANDREW:** Call the Ordering Place! We add a much-needed step to the process of requesting goods and services!

9:40: Sean finally orders a pizza with no meat...Andrew asks for sausage, which sends Sean into what appears to be an oft-repeated pizza rant:

> **SEAN:** Here's the thing...I don't eat pork, and if you get a sausage or pepperoni side and I order a cheese side, your

meat is going to encroach onto at least two of my pieces, one on each side, which essentially makes two of my pieces meat pieces, and that's topping imperialism. Get your own pizza.

9:45: Product idea: The Great Wall of Pizza™—nonstick metal topping dividers for half-and-half pizzas to protect against topping encroachment. Still no sketch ideas.

9:48: Hot dogs are discussed and I remind everyone to only eat all-beef hot dogs based on something I heard from the last guy I went on a date with, whose father worked for the USDA.

> **ANDREW:** Otherwise it's only blood vessels and rat penises, right?
>
> **ME:** Right! Wait, so if a rat's in there, his whole body would've fallen in, but you're most concerned about the penis being in there?
>
> **ANDREW:** Well, yes, if you rendered the whole body, the penis would be part of it. But it'd be a delicacy if you ate it on its own.

Shockingly, still no sketch ideas.

9:50: A conversation about expert snipers is under way. Andrew says that snipers sometimes have to account for the curvature of the earth in their shots because the bullets go so far. Jason mentions the film *American Sniper*.

JASON: Did you see that first scene when he took that guy out? He used the—

ANDREW: Ehhhh! Spoilers! I haven't seen it!

JASON: How is that a spoiler?

ANDREW: You said he snipes!

JASON: Well, yes of course he's sniping. It's called *American Sniper.* It's not gonna ruin it when you know he's sniping. The spoiler would be if he *didn't* snipe!

ANDREW: I just hate spoilers.

10:04: I have another mini-anxiety attack and Sean finally has a sketch idea.

SEAN: I heard this thing about Thomas Jefferson, how he claims that for fifty years, the sun never caught him in bed. We reenact that as if he's cheating on the sun with the moon or something.

ANDREW: Alexander Hamilton's cat was bisexual. How many presidents' cats do you think were gay?

JASON: Most of them. Does light really not penetrate a potato?

ME: That doesn't have anything to do with presidents.

JASON: I know. It has something to do with the other thing. I don't know what it is yet.

ME: What if we did something about strange presidential facts?

SEAN: Calvin Coolidge had six fingers on one hand and couldn't whistle.

ANDREW: William Howard Taft couldn't be tickled.

JASON: Ronald Reagan was a ring-tailed lemur.

ANDREW: Of course light doesn't penetrate a potato, Jason. Jesus.

10:15: Two hours in, and we don't have any usable sketch ideas, but we still think the Great Wall of Pizza is a viable product idea.

10:49: We're all watching a baby laugh hysterically at a dog eating popcorn on YouTube. Sean has ended up on a site called ToddleTales. It's as if he's gotten to the end of the internet—there were no more sites he could be on.

JASON: There should be a service for when you get to the end of the internet, called Internet Two. It's where illegal things happen and people upload Xeroxed *Cathy* comics.

11:00: At the end of the night, Sean mentions that the comic-book character Iceman recently came out as gay. Jason has an idea for a sketch where other superheroes feel like they can tell their own truths: Aquaman's a hoarder, Wonder Woman's always dreamed of being an insurance adjuster, etc. After two and a half hours, it's our only viable sketch idea. The boys leave, not really caring whether or not this has been successful because they are high and just had pizza.

All in all, I wouldn't say it was a failed experiment, though we didn't end up writing any of the stoned sketch ideas for the gonzo show.

It probably goes without saying that weed didn't facilitate a creative epiphany for me. This was now the second OFW experiment (after the sensory-deprivation tank) where I was supposed to have a creative breakthrough and didn't. Unless you consider the Great Wall of Pizza a breakthrough.

Maybe I was irredeemably blocked. Maybe I'd had a creative epiphany years before and didn't know it, and this was as good as it got. Maybe I should've been an accountant. I obviously had an affinity for spreadsheets.

I still had to find a way to unstick myself creatively, and I had no idea how to go about doing that.

On the plus side, if the OFW Project was meant to test my boundaries, well, I'd found one. I was never smoking pot again, even though it didn't have the calories of alcohol, which was always its biggest selling point for me. No high, no creative epiphany, no memorable story was worth risking the hell of a panic attack. I needed to start treating my brain with more care.

I also learned a lesson about repeating past mistakes, the lesson being that, y'know, you probably shouldn't do it. If you think you're different now or the world is different now or the bad thing won't happen again even though it happened pretty dependably before: you're not, it's not, and it will.

This message brought to you by legal weed.

Dating the Polyamorous I:

In Which I Develop an Aversion to Soccer Equipment

At this point, I was a few months and twenty first dates into my online-dating adventures, and since the beginning I'd noticed a lot of men who sent me messages described themselves as *in a relationship* or *married* in their profiles. Their missives almost always began with a disclaimer: *Once you read my profile, you may not be interested, but...* or *A lot of women run screaming when they read my profile, but let me explain...*

I'd had friends who'd been in polyamorous relationships, but it never seemed appealing to me. If you're not familiar with polyamory, you're about to be. All signs point to consensual nonmonogamous relationships being on the rise among people in their thirties and forties. Only about 5 percent of relationships are polyamorous right now, but since it's pretty much the standard among college-age daters, we can look forward to seeing more of it.

Polyamory doesn't just mean dating as many people at one time as you like, though it can mean that. How most poly couples define polyamory is that they have a primary relationship—a husband, wife, or husband- or wifelike partner—and then secondary, tertiary, and quaternary relationships depending on how ambitious/exhausted/STD-wary they are.

Up to this point, my only experience with polyamory was a couple I'd known about a decade ago, Kara and Tim, who were friends with my boyfriend at the time. They were straight out of Portland Central Casting—he was a tattooed nurse who dabbled in metallurgy and she was a sweet, Columbia Sportswear–covered brunette who worked in an after-school arts program. They were warm and funny and seemed very much in love. The first night I met them, they told me about their favorite hobby.

"We like to go to clubs together and pick out girls to play with," Kara said, grinning at Tim.

"'Play with'?" I said. "That sounds gross."

"No—she's just trying to be shocking," Tim said, fiddling with his skull ring. "Everyone knows what's what. We all get what we want out of it, including Kara."

Tim added that in the beginning, Kara was even more enthusiastic about their hobby than he was. He said he was having a little trouble keeping up with her.

At one point, she even started going out on her own and picking up women. One night, she brought home a beautiful young blonde, and they both started sleeping with her.

Kara and Tim came over for dinner a few weeks later, and while the boys were out back smoking, Kara wiped away her tears with her dinner napkin while she told me that the young blonde had moved into their bed, and Kara had been sleeping on the couch.

"How does something like that happen?" I asked. "Don't you have rules about that stuff?"

"I didn't think we needed them," she said. "I thought it was just understood."

I tried to be sympathetic, but all I could think was *There are way smarter gifts to bring home to your husband than a hot young blonde. Like a riding mower. Or an older Russian woman with a prominent ear mole. Anything but a hot young blonde, really.*

Ultimately (spoiler alert!), Kara and Tim didn't make it.

Watching this slo-mo train wreck, I concluded that polyamory was ridiculous and illogical. I was already overly anxious that my boyfriend would break up with me at any moment, either because I'd gained five pounds or because I didn't know where Kazakhstan was. I didn't need a beautiful bisexual blonde waiting in the wings for my latest fuckup. (I wasn't very secure in that relationship, if you didn't catch that.)

It also seemed impossible to me that a person wouldn't eventually fall in love with one of the secondary relationships. Old love has a very hard time competing with new lust. In a cage match between Sandwich Night with your yoga-pants-clad wife and Three-Blow-Job Tuesday with your pencil-skirt-and-stiletto-clad mistress who has no faults yet, the latter will roundhouse-kick the former in the face every time. And stilettos hurt.

So, of course, based on my experience with Kara and Tim, I ignored the e-mails from poly people.

Then I thought about it. In the most significant relationship I'd had in my life, I'd allowed myself to fall so deeply that I almost didn't survive when it ended. The pain of that loss floored me; it was, in some ways, worse than a death. At least when someone dies, you can't visit his Facebook page and see pictures of him with all his new friends at the TGI Fridays in heaven.

I mourned that relationship for longer than I was in it. So now, I thought maybe if I dated someone I knew was taken, my brain wouldn't allow me to get too attached and I would be protected from any possibility of reflooring.

The whole point of the OFW Project was to do things that I wouldn't normally do, but with at least a couple first dates a month in addition to some second and third ones, dating had totally turned into something I'd normally do. If OkCupid had a punch-card program, by this time I would've collected at least ten free men in Dockers.

This was my year to be bold and brave and not date only coders who took salsa lessons. My year to catch up. To do all the stupid shit other people got to do in their twenties. To date guys named Bodhi and learn how boring tantric sex is.[1]

Polyamory was something I couldn't picture myself doing long term, but I was definitely curious about what it would be like to be with someone who was already in a relationship. I felt like with polyamory, the pressure would be off me—there was a built-in easy out with these people, and the stakes were so much lower than in

---

[1] I don't know for sure that tantric sex is boring, but if Sting's seven-hour tantric-sex session is any indication, I'm not interested. Sex should never require an hour for lunch and two fifteen-minute compensable authorized breaks to be used at my discretion.

traditional dating. I could meet lots of people without getting all in my head with questions like *Where is this going?* and *Is he the one?* and *Where's a good place to store all my faults so he'll fall in love with me?*

If I was ever going to try polyamory, now was the time.

I'd gotten a few messages from a polyamorous married man who had seen me onstage at *Live Wire!*. His face was pixelated in his profile, since he was an IP lawyer for a very prominent startup and hadn't told anyone about his "lifestyle choice." I'd never dated anyone pixelated before, but I was willing to try. Discrimination is wrong, you guys.

He'd sent me a couple messages about how much he enjoyed *Live Wire!* but didn't make any obvious allusions to dating me, so I assumed he was just a fan of the show. This was good. Since I wasn't sure I was ready to date a polyamorous person and was merely poly-curious, I asked if he might be willing to have what I termed an "informational interview" about polyamory with me. I was shocked when he agreed.

I'm very open about all this, he wrote in an e-mail. *I mean, except with my co-workers and friends and family, but other than that...*

We agreed to meet at a pie shop in the Alberta Arts District. My favorite thing was to get a piece of banana cream and a piece of choco-late cream so I could have half of each in every bite. And since this wasn't technically a date, I could indulge in my genius pie-eating technique/gluttony at will.

Jeremy was a handsome guy—he was in his late thirties, probably six foot three, dark-haired, and very thin. He resembled Clive Owen if Clive had unnecessarily gone to Weight Watchers. He showed up looking very lawyerly in a suit, and we decided to sit outside since it was a rare sunny day.

I asked him when he and his wife had decided to become polyamorous.

"I think about...four years ago?" he answered. "We were on vacation in Thailand and we saw someone we were both interested in. I think we came to the conclusion that we should try polyamory at almost exactly the same time."

They'd tried various iterations of the poly lifestyle: they swinged (swang? swung?)[2] with other couples and tried group sex, and each had had secondary and sometimes tertiary relationships.

He was on OkCupid because his last secondary relationship had just broken up. His wife, however, had a second who was working out just fine.

"So are you just not a jealous person?" I asked.

I couldn't imagine not caring that the person I loved was in a relationship with another person. Just thinking about it made my stomach hurt. Although that could've been the pie(s).

"I've never been particularly jealous, no," he answered. "But it's not really that."

"So what is it?"

He thought about it for a second.

"It's that I'm absolutely positive that there's no one out there who

---

2 Quick clarification: Swinging is generally when couples swap partners, and it's usually fleeting and more recreational, whereas polyamory is usually defined as a more permanent situation where people become involved emotionally with other people. But of course there's some crossover. Polyamory and swinging, as you can imagine, don't have hard-and-fast rules. But there are other things involved that are hard and fast. *Bam!* Sex joke!

loves her as much as I do, and she's absolutely positive that there's no one out there who loves me as much as she does."

"So you can cheat on each other because you love each other so much?" I asked.

"It's not cheating if you agree to it," he said. "And yes. There's no reason for me to be jealous of men who have no chance of being what I am to her."

How foreign. And strangely romantic.

It seemed like Jeremy's biggest issue was finding the right mix in a second. A secondary relationship for him was just that—secondary. But it wasn't just about sex. He wanted real intimacy; it just needed to take up less time and mental space than his primary relationship. The problem was that once he and a second got involved emotionally, she would inevitably become dissatisfied with sharing him and want him to leave his wife. This had happened to him three times already.

This is the cost, I imagine, of being on the bleeding edge of relationship technology. His brain had grown accustomed to the new rules, but he kept meeting women who either hadn't yet acclimated to them or had agreed to the terms and conditions without asking themselves if they were truly prepared for the consequences. (Those of us with Apple products who received a forced U2 song can relate.)

"I'd probably respond the same way if I became emotionally involved with someone," I said. "I'm not sure I'd be very good at the poly thing."

"Maybe not." He smiled. "But it's working out pretty well for me."

We talked for a little longer while he finished his lunch and I pretended not to be able to finish my two pieces of pie. (Acting!)

When we parted, he practically speed-walked away from the table.

Clearly he wasn't interested in actually dating me, which was probably for the best since I had my doubts about how well I'd do as a second.

Then, a few days later, I ran across Joe's profile. He was adorable and seemed to have a sense of humor, which was rare on OkCupid. After lots of hovering over his Like button, I finally clicked it, and he wrote me the standard disclaimer. *I assume you've read my profile, but just to be sure, I need you to know I'm in a pretty unique situation...*

I knew.

After a few e-mails back and forth, Joe (aka first date #21) and I met for drinks at a pool hall. Dressed in cargo shorts and a T-shirt (the summer uniform for Portland dads), he was taller and more muscular than he looked in his pictures, which was the opposite of how things usually worked. He was probably about six feet, two hundred and twenty pounds, with a healthy tan and a sweet, boyish face. He was Canadian, which I found adorable due to either my love for Justin Trudeau or my affinity for tuques. We played a couple of games, then went to an Irish pub for more cocktails.

He got a text.

"Do you have to go?" I asked. I didn't know what the rules were.

"Oh, no," he said. "She's at home with someone, so I have to be out for at least another couple hours or so."

"Cool," I said nonchalantly so he wouldn't know that inside I was totally *Holy shit*–ing.

If I were part of a polyamorous couple, there would be no dates in our shared house. I don't want some basic bitch's butt on the midcentury couch we picked out together at that little shop on Hawthorne, the one with the store cat. That was a good day and her ass ruined it. (Reason #836 that I'm probably not cut out for polyamory.)

"So how long have you been doing this poly thing?" I asked.

"I think a few months now?" he said. "It was my wife's suggestion."

"Wow," I said.

"Is that surprising?" he asked.

"I think I have this idea that a lot of husbands cajole their wives into swinging," I said.

"Nah," he said. "It was all her. She's younger than me. I think there are still oats she wants to sow."

"And you're cool with that?"

"I think it'll be good for us," he said.

"In what way?"

"I don't know," he said. "I think if she meets a lot of guys, it'll make her realize that everyone has faults, not just me. Maybe she'll love me more."

It was the sweetest reason to agree to allow your wife to sleep with a lot of men I'd ever heard.

He said the poly life had been going well for them. Exceptionally well for her, fairly well for him. This was, apparently, a trend. He and his wife knew a few other poly couples, and almost across the board, the women got significantly more action than the men.

"That makes sense to me," I said.

"Why?" he asked.

"Because men are generally happy to get sex however it comes, whereas women would tend not to trust a man who says he's in an open marriage."

"Huh," he said. "Do you trust me?"

"I do," I said.

"Why?"

"Because you just told me that your wife gets way more action than you," I said. "If you were lying, you'd say the opposite."

We sat and talked until he was cleared to go home. Continuing the dating trend I'd been experiencing for about six months, we didn't have a lot of shared interests—he worked in medical IT and liked to camp (super-ick), and I'm reasonably sure he golfed. But he was cute and refreshingly unassuming and I enjoyed spending time with him. If he hadn't been married, he would've fit into the category of People I Should Sleep With for a While Until One of Us Starts Getting Too Attached, at Which Point the Other Will Quietly Disappear. But since he was married, he fit into the category of People I Should Sleep With for a While Until... Their Wives Say They Can't Anymore? I Don't Know How This Works.

I assumed he'd tell me.

At the end of the date, he walked me to my car and we leaned on my Civic and kissed. I don't kiss on a lot of first dates, but when you're auditioning to be someone's second or third, things tend to move faster. There's no reason to go through the regular dating rigmarole since this is not going to be a story you tell your grandkids.

Joe's kissing style wasn't my cup of tea (very wet, like he was kissing me with the inside of his lips, which made me wonder if someone had once told him his kisses were too dry and he overcorrected), but there was definitely enough sexual chemistry to pique my curiosity.

With Joe, I'd come to expand my horizons, but, weirdly, I stayed for the intimacy.

After our second date, Joe came back to my place, and Things Happened.[3]

After a highly successful rolling-around session wherein we never even bothered to get fully into my bed, we were lying on top of my comforter giggling quietly and talking, and Joe did the most surprising thing: He took my hand. And as we continued talking, he softly ran his fingers up and down my forearm as if he'd been doing it for years.

We'd just had what was definitely casual sex, but this physical act was such a convincing simulacrum of actual intimacy that it was jarring.

And after thinking about it, I decided it made sense.

He was married, so of course he was comfortable with physical and emotional intimacy. He'd agreed to a lifetime of it. With someone else, sure, but that's really splitting hairs.

We lay there for about a half an hour that night, his hands running over my arms, my back, his fingers running through my hair, and we talked about his marriage, my work, and how he'd become so skilled with his tongue. (He'd read a book, it turns out, called *She Comes First*, which I will tell you, men, was *much appreciated*. I mean, I own the equipment and sometimes even I'm befuddled by it.)

Then he started talking about his work, and I was mostly listening to him, but part of me was so distracted by this unexpected tenderness and the softness of his hands that I had a hard time focusing on the mechanics of how to build a fully integrated enterprise platform.

This was exactly what I was looking for. This kind of intimacy. This

---

3   We did it.

kind of touch. I wanted it so much that the more my arms tingled, the more my chest ached.

Except for the niggling details of him being married and us not having anything in common, it was perfect.

After about thirty minutes of the best afterglow of my life, Joe got up and got dressed in the dark, something I'm sure he'd become good at in the past few months.

When he was ready to go, he sat on the bed and kissed me.

"Is this awkward for you?" he asked. "Are you okay?"

I was a little shocked. Those are two thorny questions that have a high probability of not getting the response one is hoping for. It wasn't awkward and I was okay, but it was lovely to be asked.

It turned out that yet another thing Joe was adept at was having difficult conversations.

His decision to become polyamorous had forced him to have so many of them with his wife that he'd become a pro. This was incredibly refreshing in the "Let's hang out sometime," impossible-to-tell-whether-you're-dating-or-not-due-to-imprecise-language Portland dating scene.

I started taking advantage of the skills Joe offered on a fairly regular basis at the same time I was dating other people. Sometimes we'd meet at my house, sometimes at a bar.

One night he called me and said his wife was on a date and did I want to come over.

To his house? With his five-year-old twin daughters there?

That was a whole different ball of wax. Or can of worms. Or house with a family that could come spilling out.

I have no issues when it comes to polyamory—adults can do whatever they want with their bodies and hearts and marriages. But when you bring children into the mix, I'm definitely uncomfortable.

But what if Joe were gay? Would I say, *I'm okay with you marrying a man as long as you don't bring kids into it?* I'm either down or not down, right?

I decided that if I was okay with polyamory, I had to be okay with it even if kids were involved.

I agreed to meet him at his house after his girls went to bed.

As I was getting ready, I imagined what his house would look like. Who made most of the decorating choices, him or his wife? And what did he do for his at-home dates? Would I walk in to candles and wine? And would they be candles his wife had bought at Bath and Body Works on $8.95 Candle Day?

I walked through the front door and was immediately bombarded with family stuff: Photos of all of them in matching denim shirts and khakis taken by a professional photographer. Video games and toys everywhere. A miniature easel and whiteboard with a drawing of a little girl in the sun with flowers coming out of her head.

Come *on*.

It was like she knew Daddy had a date and she wanted her to be racked with guilt and question the entire concept of nontraditional relationships.

Little shit.

"Have you had other dates here?" I asked.

"Sure," he replied. "My wife does it all the time."

It reminded me of those teen movies where one kid has been suckered by a group of ne'er-do-wells into coming along on some ill-fated shenanigans, like breaking into a public pool or killing a hobo. Invariably, the new kid asks, "Are you sure this is cool?" And the leader of the gang who will later be impaled by a fence post says, "Sure. We do it all the time."

I rocked from foot to foot as we chatted quietly for a little while.

"Where are the girls' rooms?" I whispered.

"Oh, they're downstairs," he said. "But you don't have to whisper. They sleep really soundly."

Do you have that in writing somewhere? I don't want to get nitpicky, but this could get life-alteringly uncomfortable for all of us.

Since I wanted to get out of any common areas of the house, we moved to the guest room and started kissing. Right after we pushed his daughter's soccer gear off the bed.

Hello, boner-killer.

Joe said he had to leave the door slightly open just in case one of his daughters woke up—he had to be able to hear them.

Really? What if we were in flagrante and one of them came up and gently pushed the door open without us hearing a thing? I imagined it happening, the door slowly opening to reveal a daughter, who my brain decided to picture as Cindy Lou Who. The giant, disappointed eyes. The antennae.

Antennae or not, I didn't want to do that to a kid. I didn't want to be the reason her father had to explain what *polyamory* means. I also didn't have the money to pay for a lifetime of therapy for a five-year-old. That's hundreds of thousands of dollars, probably. I'd rather cover her college tuition.

Problem was, I definitely wanted to have sex with Joe that night. He had the kind of skill that if you thought about having sex with him, you couldn't get the idea of it out of your head until you had it, like really good sushi or the right to vote. Plus, wasn't I *supposed* to be stepping out of my comfort zone? I got up and pushed the door closed as much as I could while still leaving enough space so that Joe could hear his kids.

His *kids*.

He kissed me. I kissed him back. He kissed my neck. I looked at the door. He pulled my sweater down and kissed my breast. I thought about how quiet a five-year-old's footfall was on carpeted steps. They were like cats, only bigger. He pulled my skirt down. I pulled it up and pulled off my underwear—that way if I had to stand up quickly, I'd appear fully clothed with only one boob out, which seems slightly less traumatizing for a child than Dad and a naked lady.

He went down on me. This was perfect. It was quiet and still gave me a great view of the door. It was also by far the fastest way to an orgasm—when it came to power and accuracy, his tongue was like a wet, soft Tomahawk missile. Which would be of no use to the Defense Department but was quite useful for me.

I allowed myself to close my eyes for just long enough to get where I needed to go while keeping eagle...ears on the stairwell. (*Do eagles have good ears? Their heads are completely smooth. That's weird. Note to self: Look that up right after you stop having sex with polyamorous married dudes with kids.*) I came, and then I did everything I could to get Joe off as quickly as possible while still checking for ominous shadows in the doorway. It was like watching two people have sex in a horror film, when you're just waiting for the killer to come and use one whale spear to turn them into a sexy shish kebab. Except that I was one of the two people, and the killer was a five-year-old wielding a Polyamory Barbie (now with two Kens!). Thankfully, she never showed.

When we were done, I put my boob back in its holster and pulled on my underwear—no afterglow this time.

Joe kissed me at the door and said he'd text me later to make sure I got home okay.

I got in my car and knew immediately.

The devil-may-care, try-everything-once attitude I was attempting to cultivate in myself had, for the first time, steered me wrong.

I thought about all the times when I was a kid that my parents probably thought I was sleeping soundly, but I wasn't. Conversations I'd heard, laughter that wafted up to my bedroom from their gatherings, strange silences that I knew held something I shouldn't know about.

Even though Joe and I hadn't gotten caught, I hated thinking that I might have been one of those memories for his girls.

Was that orgasm worth it? I could've just as easily given one to myself. I'm very good at it.

So far, I'd had some great experiences, some solidly so-so ones, and one that almost made me see stars from physical pain (the Brazilian). But this was the first one I truly regretted and that I felt had, ever so slightly, turned me into a worse person instead of a better one.

I still enjoyed spending time with Joe and thought I'd probably see him again.

Just no more at-home dates with polyamorous men. Too messy, and too much of a chance that you'll come into contact with the people they actually love.

As it turns out, some boundaries are good.

Dating the Polyamorous II:

In Which I Learn Who the Boss Is, and It's Not Judith Light

As I was dating Joe, I continued to trade messages with Jeremy. He would periodically check in with me on OkCupid chat.

> JEREMY: Hey! How's it going?
>
> ME: Okay. But I'm getting frustrated. Why doesn't anyone have a sense of humor?
>
> JEREMY: It's Portland. Everyone's in their safe space.
>
> ME: True. I'm in mine right now. (It's the Ikea cafeteria.) How's by you?
>
> JEREMY: I'm okay. I'm with this girl who wants me to pee on her, though.

ME: Holy shit. What'd you say?[1]

JEREMY: I already had sex with her in front of her boyfriend at his request. I feel like I've done my due diligence with this person.

ME: Come on. You did not do that.

JEREMY: He had a voyeur thing.

ME: What was it like?

JEREMY: It was like fucking, but I was just more conscious of what my gut looked like from the side.

ME: Now you know what it's like for women to have sex.

JEREMY: Touché. Anyway, he's her boyfriend...he should pee on her. Not me.

ME: See? If I didn't know you, I wouldn't know that rule.

JEREMY: Yeah, you're welcome.

His sex life was so varied and fascinating, I couldn't look away. We started talking about sex more often, and because I didn't think we'd ever see each other again, I felt totally free to say things that it'd take me much longer to reveal to someone I was dating. During one conversation, he said that his girlfriend had asked him to tell her what to do to another man via text, in real time.

ME: That sounds complicated.

---

1   This is one of those fetishes in which I get caught up in the logistics. Where does one get peed on? Do you always have to have sex in the shower? And then later, when you pee in the shower for convenience, does that turn you on? For a golden-showers person, is peeing on yourself like masturbation? *I have so many questions.*

JEREMY: Nah. It's just sexting, except there's someone physically there taking your place.

ME: So it's like sex by proxy. Seems like you got the short
end of that stick.

JEREMY: It was fun. I like dominating her.

There was a lag in the conversation as I typed and deleted and retyped
my next comment.

ME: I've always fantasized about being dominated.

And another, shorter lag.

JEREMY: I could do that for you. I'm good at it.

This was a wrinkle I wasn't expecting. I had been dating a lot, but
clearly I was still a total amateur at deciphering whether someone
was interested in me.

ME: I thought you weren't interested in me in that way.

JEREMY: No! I just thought that when you said you wouldn't
be good at polyamory, you meant you weren't into trying it
with me.

A wave of adrenaline washed over me from the tip of my head all the
way down my torso. It crashed right around my vagina.

The idea of actually being dominated by someone after thinking
about it for so long left me almost breathless.

Like Sally in *When Harry Met Sally,* my fantasy fodder has been the same for my whole adult life: I'm a secretary and my boss expects more of me than just dictation.[2] I'm not sure why I chose secretary, but I type about ninety words per minute, so if I'm going to fantasize about a job in the clerical milieu, that one makes the most sense. Also, naughty secretary sounds much sexier than naughty stenographer. But I digress.

In the fantasy, my generic, slightly blurry boss pushes me up against his giant dark wood desk, shoves his hand down a pair of much sexier panties than I generally wear, and forces me to do things. He's holding something over my head—figuratively—so I have to do whatever he says. I say no initially and try to fight him off, but once we're in the middle of it, I start to like it.

Oftentimes it'll include one of his male colleagues who just happens to be in the office after hours. Maybe they're working on a project together. Something businessy?

Nothing derails a sex fantasy faster than trying to figure out the details. Like, what's he holding over me? Is it just that I really need the job, or have I been embezzling money? And what kind of company is it, anyway? No one has secretaries anymore. He must be really old if he can't send his own e-mails.

In any case, I've had this same fantasy for years, and it's worked for me over and over again.

It's pretty inconvenient to be a feminist and have a constant fantasy of being overtaken by two men.

According to *Psychology Today,* one explanation for why women have rape fantasies is "sexual blame avoidance." Because so many

---

2   More like "*dick*-tation," amiright? I'll see myself out.

women have guilt about their sexuality, a scene in which they're taken against their will allows them to escape any sense of culpability, so they can enjoy their fantasy guilt-free.

That wasn't me.

Thankfully, the same study also turned up a different explanation for what appears to be disempowering daydreams: certain women, for whatever reason, are the opposite of those women who have guilt around sex. They're so open to sexual experiences that they can have fantasies that go beyond the bounds of what is considered sexually appropriate behavior without any emotional repercussions.

I think because I started having sex so late in life, I'm far more open to divergent sexual experiences than a lot of my friends. I've always felt that my late start gave me free rein for a couple reasons. One was that once I tried sex and realized how much I loved it, I felt cheated, like the universe owed me a *lot* of sex and I was going to do whatever I could to get it. The other was that I figured if you held on to your virginity for long enough, you could remain a virgin emeritus for the rest of your life, avoiding judgment from friends, lovers, and maybe even God, who I haven't yet decided exists (I figure that, unless I get hit by a bus, I have about twenty years to figure that out).

So at the moment Jeremy made his offer, my hesitation about indulging in my fantasy with him wasn't about crossing some self- or culturally imposed line of sexual norms; it was more about whether I thought I would actually enjoy it. Did I actually want to be dominated in the real world, or would it make me feel truly subjugated instead of pseudo-subjugated?

And who was this guy, really? I'd never talked to his wife. Maybe he wasn't married anymore because his wife was cut up into stew meat in his freezer.

When you have anxiety, it's sometimes hard to differentiate between excitement and trepidation. This was obviously a little of both.

He said we should meet for a drink to see if we might want to meet for something else.

I wanted to. But it was a lot at once.

Then again, the OFW Project had brought me this thing that I theoretically wanted. I continued to be curious about polyamory and about what it felt like to be dominated. Wasn't it my job to sally forth into the unknown in spite of my fears? Wasn't that the whole point of this year? To take these offers from the God of Questionable Sexual Choices just as I would've in my twenties if I hadn't hated my body at the time?

I swallowed hard and agreed to meet Jeremy that evening at a new Japanese fusion place near my house.

It was a cold, industrial space with polished cement floors, bright red tables, and matching bright red wooden chairs. My dread ball started growing in my chest about an hour before I arrived at the bar, and when I got there I wondered if the décor was the universe trying to wave a red flag at me.

We hugged when we saw each other, leaning in gingerly and doing the upper-torso, two-pat, I-don't-know-you-that-well-so-don't-make-it-weird special.

He was more attractive than I remembered. More put together. Had he done something to himself, or was I just remembering him wrong?

We sat down and talked about horribly boring shit for a couple minutes to fill the space. I had revealed a *lot* to this man I'd met only once, and I was having some trouble reconciling those two things, the same way I had with Text Guy.

My sake cocktail arrived with his bourbon. This would help.

"How are things going with your wife?" I asked, shifting the conversation to comfortable territory we'd covered online.

"They're fine," he said, shaking his glass to cool down his whiskey. "She seems happy with this guy and I'm happy for her. But sometimes it's hard when one of us has a second and the other doesn't."

"I'm sure," I said. "She's probably not as available as you'd like."

"Yeah, and we're having less sex," he said as he took a swig of his bourbon.

"Is that normal?" I asked.

"Sometimes," he said. "When it's new."

"That must be hard," I said.

"Nah," he said. "Kinda goes with the territory."

As my cocktail kicked in and the subject matter got more interesting, my dread ball was shrinking as my curiosity grew. We talked about his relationships, my dates, what I knew about polyamory, and how that jibed with his reality. Eventually we started talking about his stranger sexual encounters, like spending an evening in a sex club with his wife and three other people.

"What was that like?" I asked.

"It was definitely difficult to navigate physically," he replied. "It was about two to three more people than would be my ideal."

"I don't think I could even do a threesome," I said.

"Why?" he asked.

"It would be like one long sixty-nine session," I said.

He laughed. "In what way?" he asked.

"Well, sixty-nine-ing can be nice," I replied. "But the entire time, you're trying to concentrate on giving the other person pleasure while also trying to concentrate on what's happening to you. As in most cases of multitasking, I think both experiences can suffer."

"That's more thought than I'd ever give to that," he said. "But it makes sense."

By now my breathing was less shallow and the knots in my stomach were coming untied. Each story made him more intriguing and, weirdly, sort of admirable in a Meriwether Lewis–of–the–sexual–world kinda way.

I got another drink, and my questions to Jeremy got bolder, as did my admissions.

As with what felt like almost every single person I'd met online, I didn't have a lot in common with Jeremy, but this was different somehow. I hadn't had much in common with the other guys because I didn't understand how to use Java as a server-side language for back-end development. I didn't have much in common with Jeremy because I'd never had a fivesome.

But unlike with those other men, with Jeremy I was actually interested in the things that made us different, and the idea of him dominating me kept creeping into my head as we spoke.

After a couple of hours in the bar, we moved to the picnic tables outside, where we sat on the same side of one of the tables, facing out.

"Can I kiss you?" he asked.

I squinted at him, half pretending to be wary. Because I was half wary.

"Sure," I said, grinning.

We started to kiss, and at one point he grabbed the back of my head in a way that made me immediately think about making bad choices.

He suggested we go back to my place.

I had some misgivings about this. My vagina didn't.

He followed me to my house, which was only about five minutes away.

It was late, so we walked quietly to the old pool house in the back that my roommate and I had been using as a sort of love shack. Jeremy and I made out some more in the doorway, him pressing up against me.

"So, if we were to do this domination thing, how would that work?" I asked.

"We'd just do it," he said breathlessly.

"Shouldn't we have a safe word, just in case I don't like it?"

"Oh, right," he said, backing off. "Of course. Do you have one?"

"No," I said. "I've never needed one before."

"Okay, so it should just be something you wouldn't normally say," he whispered while kissing my neck. "Like, it definitely shouldn't be *no*, because *no* might be part of the fantasy. It should be a word that you have no reason to say, like *pineapple*."

"Okay, let's make it *pineapple*," I said, pulling him in.

"You sure?" he said. "A safe word is a kind of personal thing."

He was right. I'm a writer. I couldn't just appropriate someone else's safe word.

My mind went blank.

"I don't know. What if I choose one that breaks the mood?" I said.

"Like what?" he asked, clearly less in the mood.

"I don't know...*grandma* or *impotence.*"

"Can you not mention impotence right now?" he said, rubbing his eyes a little.

"See?"

He left to pee while I thought about it a minute. "I got it," I said when he returned. "*Safe word.*"

"Really?" he said.

"Yeah. That way, you'll stop immediately. If I picked a different one, there might be a minute where you're like, *Was that supposed to be the safe word, or was it* grandma?"

He grabbed my face and held it.

"Stop saying *grandma,*" he said, smiling, then he kissed me hard.

"Okay," I said between kisses as he led me into the pool house.

We got to the bed.

"You really want me to do this?" he asked.

"Please," I said.

He pushed me down onto the bed. I gasped a little. I was immediately, insanely aroused.

He told me to get on my knees. And then he started ordering me around in earnest.

Normally, I'm not a fan of bossy people. In the real world, I tend to bristle when anyone tells me what to do or how to do it.

But in the bedroom, surrendering my will to someone else wasn't just a relief, it was wildly hot. The bossier Jeremy got, the more I quivered.

And he got very bossy. Not bossy enough that I needed to use my safe word, *safe word,* but still.

This acting-out-the-opposite-role-in-the-bedroom theme comes up a lot in the BDSM (bondage/discipline/sadomasochism) world. It's said that the more dominant people are in their work and home lives, the more submissive they want to be sexually; it's a relief and a vacation from themselves to let go.

Some people have even posited that for truly bossy people—people who subjugate others to their will all the time—being a sexual submissive is a way to do penance.

That definitely wasn't me. The only power one has at a public radio show is the ability to get someone a free tote bag.

Funny thing is, even though I was submitting, I was also still sort of the boss because I'd asked Jeremy to dominate me. That's the strange circular logic of the dominant/submissive relationship.

During our pool-house session, Jeremy acted out the perfect amount of dominance for me, shedding the bossiness when it came time to make sure all my needs were met and that orgasms were had by all.

Afterward, there wasn't a lot of afterglow, but there was a lot of sweat and even more laughing. I had surprised myself and I think he'd done the same.

"Was that okay?" he asked, not in the "How was it for you?" sense, more in a "How weird was that for you on a scale of one to infinity?" kind of way.

It had been the most incendiary sexual encounter I'd ever had. Not a speck of tenderness or emotional intimacy, just raw, unfettered sexuality. With a guy who—following what seemed to be the trend of the year—I wasn't that interested in emotionally.

And I really enjoyed it.

"Yeah," I replied. "It was kinda great."

"Well, I enjoyed the hell out of it," he said. "I hope we can do it again."

He got dressed while I lounged on the bed and replayed some of the better moments from our session. He leaned down and kissed me before leaving to go home to his wife.

I stayed in the pool house that night. I left the doors open to the cool night air. Sometimes Portland takes an early turn to fall. It's impatient, maybe. I can relate.

Days after that encounter, I was still fantasizing about it—something I'd never done with any other partner. So I saw him again.

We probably saw each other three times in the next six weeks, the third time at a hipster hotel in Southeast Portland. I adore hotels and was excited at the prospect of actually being the mistress in the hotel even though we totally had permission.

We had sex twice that night, but Jeremy wasn't feeling particularly dominant so it was only semi-hot and didn't have the earth-shattering impact our first encounter had.

He had to leave afterward (he and his wife had a rule that they couldn't have overnights without special permission) but he told me that I could stay as long as I wanted to.

I enjoyed the sex, but I also couldn't wait to have a hotel room to myself. Cable. An ice machine. Full minibar access. I was very excited by the prospect of cuddling with myself.

When he left, I fell back into the kajillion-thread-count sheets and watched cable while eating M&M's.

Jeremy and I texted each other for a while after that, but we never saw each other again.

Even though it ended with a whimper (well, two bangs, then a whimper), I was grateful I'd met him.

One reason people date is to discover what they like and don't like.

He taught me something I liked. A *lot*.

The dating portion of the OFW Project had felt pointless to me because of all the failure, but this was a case where spending time with a man I would definitely not end up with was perfectly fine. More than fine. Knowing that he wasn't the man for me was exactly what allowed me to ask him for something I couldn't have asked for otherwise. (I'd love to say I'm more evolved than this, but being honest about any perceived freakiness is a million times easier when there is zero at stake.) So now I knew it was possible for me to ask without being mortified or rejected. And now I knew what to add to my list of things to look for in a partner: bossy AF, but only sexually.

I was also learning that, when it came to sexuality, my curiosity beat out my anxiety almost every time. In this one category, I was starting to feel a little brave. Would it have been better if my bravery manifested itself as putting my body in front of a bullet meant for one of my comrades or running into a burning building to save a family of four? Sure. But we play the hand we're dealt. And some of us were dealt those naked-lady cards.

Jeremy friended me on Facebook a couple months after we dated and we stayed in touch that way.

A year and a half after I saw him for the last time, he got a divorce. His wife had fallen in love with her second and left him.

I really don't think they've worked out the glitches in polyamory yet. You may want to wait until polyamory 2.0 is released to try it.

Build-Your-Own-Burrito Night at the

Sex Club:

Wherein I Am Disappointed by Public Sex and Tortillas

No NUDITY AT THE BUFFET.

When you're in an establishment and you see this sign, you know you're probably outside your comfort zone.

My comfort zone was somewhere in Utah, perhaps, when I spent an evening at Club Sesso in downtown Portland in month nine of my Year and a Half–Ish of Activities That Lessened My Scaredy-Cat Tendencies.

Sesso (which is now, tragically, closed) was billed as "Portland's Premier Swingers Club."

The club was licensed by Ron Jeremy, America's most trusted name in on-camera intercourse.[1] "The swinging lifestyle in Portland

---

1   If you're not familiar with him, Ron Jeremy is America's best-known porn star, having done more than seventeen hundred pornographic films, includ-

and Southwest Washington has wanted an upscale erotic-lifestyle club for several years," the website claimed, and Club Sesso had "answered that demand."

The thing is, I'd lived in Portland for about eighteen years, and I'd never heard anyone demand anything like that. A seat warmer for a unicycle? You bet. Cruelty-free mustache wax? Absolutely. But no one had ever looked at me over her gluten-free barbecued tempeh sliders and said, "Y'know what this town really needs? An upscale erotic-lifestyle club."

Nonetheless, we had one.

I'd heard about this place from a friend who had taken a meeting with Mr. Jeremy in the club. She told a story about watching him eat pasta and then sign a contract with his right hand while he fingered a woman with his left. She may have made it up, but it sounded like a pretty Ron Jeremy thing to do.

I never imagined I'd actually see the inside of Sesso until I was having a conversation with Joe in bed one night after we'd been seeing each other for about a month. He was telling me about a group of polyamorous mothers his wife was in, women who would get together and chat about the challenges and frustrations of their lifestyle. I was fascinated.

"So she knows enough of them to have a group?" I said. "God, I'd love to talk to them."

"You should," he said. "But if you really want to see what the poly lifestyle is like, you should come to Sesso."

---

ing *Orgazmo, Big Butt Cowgirl Pinups,* and *The Great American Squirt-Off* (1 and 2). I am not making these titles up.

"Oh, no," I said. "I don't think I need to do that."

"Why not?" he asked. "Aren't you supposed to be doing things that you wouldn't normally do?"

"Yeah, sure. But that seems excessive."

"Okay," he said. "It's your deal."

Yes, I was incredibly curious about what Sesso might be like, but the last time I'd done something I wasn't completely comfortable with—going to Joe's house while his kids were home—it hadn't gone well. I hadn't mentioned that to Joe; I'd just told him that I didn't want to have any more at-home dates and he understood.

"Do you have to have sex there?" I asked.

He laughed. "Jesus. No. Some people just go and sit at the bar all night. There's also a pretty decent buffet."

"You're shitting me," I said.

"Not that I'm aware of."

I looked up the website on my phone. It mentioned the buffet.

"Okay," I said. "We're going."

There was something about the fact that it had a buffet that immediately calmed my nerves. Things can only get so dark and salacious when there are chafing dishes and sneeze guards nearby.

That being said, as the day approached, I got a little sweaty as I pictured myself at a fully naked, un-Cinemax-ified version of the party scene in *Eyes Wide Shut*, standing just far enough away to avoid being splattered by bodily fluids and taking notes for my column.

I felt pre-humiliated.

It wasn't the fact that it was a sex club that freaked me out the most, it was that it was a club...a place where people go to meet other people. I'm not good with social situations, especially ones where people might be wearing assless chaps and asking me if they can place something of theirs in one of my orifices.

Once I knew it was a done deal, though, my apprehension was joined by what I'm pretty sure was excitement. (I don't feel it very often, so it was either that or gas.) I knew this was likely to be an evening fraught with dicey personal interactions for me, but I'm also fascinated as hell by human sexuality in all its forms, and having an escort who had been there before was surprisingly comforting.

I told my mother this at our weekly dinner.

"You don't have to worry about it, Mom," I said. "Joe's totally been to a sex club before."

"Doesn't help," my mother said. "Might've just made it worse."

She was not a fan of the idea of me going to a sex club, but my mother was otherwise surprisingly cool with my ridiculous escapades. She is a product of the sixties, but not the hippie ones. She had been a stewardess and an army officer's wife, and I think my parents skipped the sexual revolution to attend some really fun cocktail parties. So although my OFW field trips were often things she wouldn't do herself in a million years, she wanted me to be happy and less tightly wound, so she supported me.

"We're going on fetish night," I said.

"Oh Jesus," she replied, taking another swig of her sangria spritzer.

Joe and I had decided to go to the club on fetish night because we figured it was likely to be a lot more interesting than a standard weekend night. The website said fetish clothes were encouraged, so I wore the closest thing I had—a simple black blouse with a velvet pencil skirt that laced all the way up the back with a satin bow. Joe actually wore pants instead of cargo shorts, so I knew this was a special occasion.

I felt exactly like I had the night I went to see a Missing Persons concert in high school and tried to dress new wave–y and everyone could tell I'd never smoked cloves before, except at Sesso, instead of being worried that everyone would know I was square, I was worried everyone would know that I had never tried anal and had utterly failed at the reverse cowgirl the one time I tried it.

Before we entered the club, we were asked to sign an extremely long form.

"What is this?" I whispered to Joe.

"It essentially says that you know what you're getting into and that you won't sue them if you're traumatized by what you see or do," he said.

"Aw," I said.

"What?" he asked.

"It's just so romantic," I said.

My hands were cold and tingly. The waiver didn't help to assuage my nervousness.

I took a deep breath.

Joe touched the small of my back as we walked in and then leaned into me. "We can go whenever you want," he said. "Just say the word."

The door opened and the pumping techno music that had been muffled blasted us just as the disco lights hit us.

I was surprised and relieved to find that it looked just like any other club with largely the standard clientele, aside from a few folks in S & M garb sprinkled around. There was a shiny black bar to our left and a very small dance floor to our right. The only tip-off that this might have been a sex club, aside from the one guy at the bar fondling his girlfriend's breasts, were the torture stations. To the right of the dance floor, there were two huge black Xs, each about six feet tall, for people to shackle their dates to while they tickled, spanked, whipped, licked, slapped, or spoke to them in a mildly annoyed tone about their inability to file their taxes on time. That is something you don't see at, say, a Dave and Buster's.

Oh, and there were giant TVs playing hard-core porn. Everywhere.

BDSM has gone somewhat mainstream with the success of the Harry Potter of Watered-Down and Mildly Rapey Bondage book *Fifty Shades of Grey*, but if you're unfamiliar with it, it's very important to make clear that everything that was happening to the men and women in the club, even the ones who were tied up, was completely consensual.[2]

This night, the featured fetish was *shibari*.

Shibari, meaning "to tie" in Japanese, is an ancient form of erotic rope bondage that originated in fifteenth-century Japan as *hojojutsu*, the martial art of restraining captives. It's evolved into an erotic art in which people use complex knots and rigging to create beautiful geometric shapes and patterns on and around a person's body while restraining it, often suspending him or her in midair. The riggers use the ropes to move the person's body into positions that highlight its natural curves and then torture the individual in subtle ways that increase sexual anticipation.

---

2   The BDSM community is pretty strict about communication and consent—giving it and getting it. And if all the recent sexual-harassment allegations are any indication, they should be sending men and women in bondage gear and assless chaps to give workshops on both of those subjects at every corporation in America. (I'm only half kidding here.)

Some *shibari* practitioners even position the knots on pressure points, similar to shiatsu or acupuncture.

I know.

In Portland, even our fetishes are artisanal.

From the balcony of the second floor of the club, Joe and I watched a man take at least twenty minutes to tie a woman up using *shibari*. She stood in the middle of the dance floor below us, blindfolded and naked, suspended from a rope that bound her wrists as he slowly pulled an inch-wide rope across and around her body. He took special care to pull the rope slowly across her nipples and between her legs. They clearly knew each other well, and every move he made was painstaking, purposeful, and strangely affectionate. He stopped every few minutes to whisper in her ear.

She seemed to be in a state of excruciating anticipation.

It made me wish they offered spectators earphones, like on museum and zoo tours:

As the rigger, or top, places the rope on the body of the model, or bottom, she often finds herself in what's called a sub space, a trancelike state some people refer to as "rope drunk." This rigger has just whispered, "You're such a good little sub," to his model. Now, please move on to television number seven, where we'll be discussing the film On Golden Blonde.

Shibari was happening on our floor as well. There was a long bar to our left with patrons seated in front of it with drinks, but instead of a bartender and a wall of bottles behind it, there were two queen mattresses on the floor. A naked man stood on one mattress rigging a thick rope that suspended his girlfriend horizontally, like a sexy hammock. The other mattress featured a man tending to two dangling women who were horizontally stacked on top of each other like sexual Jenga pieces. There was pretty much nowhere you could look without seeing some form of sex act or knot-tying that was outside the typical merit-badge categories.

It was overwhelming.

I turned away from the bar and saw a man standing near the action dressed like a football coach—blue polo shirt, Dockers—wearing a lanyard around his neck with the letters *DM*. He appeared to be surveying the action. I had seen more guys with DM tags on the lower floor, and I was curious as to what they did. I wanted to ask him, but...

Here's a thing about me: I don't talk to strangers. I have such a strong fear of rejection and such an aversion to bothering people that aside from waiters, bartenders, and checkout people, I never approach anyone I don't know.

But the magical thing about the OFW Project was that having to write a column about these experiences somehow emboldened me and distanced me from my anxiety. Even though my column was just about my own experience, I somehow felt like a journalist studying my own life, and that fact gave me permission to talk to this stranger, even though he had no idea why I was doing it. I also thought that talking to him might distract me from the surfeit of sex acts going on around me so I could have a little time to fucking acclimate myself.

I walked over to the DM.

"What does *DM* stand for?" I yelled over the music.

"Dungeon monitor," he answered.

"What do you do?" I asked.

"It's our job to monitor the play to ensure that no one gets hurt and that everyone's following the house rules."

I learned that DMs are trained in BDSM safety practices and first aid, and they have absolute authority—if the DM says it's over, it's over. This particular DM had been volunteering at parties and fetish nights since the eighties and trained people in fetishes like *shibari* and boot play.[3]

"Have you ever seen anyone get hurt?" I asked.

"Sure. I've seen people get cut too deeply during knife play or drop ten feet to the ground during rope play and break bones. It can get ugly but it happens very rarely, because we're here."

One of the things the DMs were doing that night, he explained, was quizzing riggers about the weight rating on their rings and carabiners to make sure that they could suspend the subs safely.

My conversation with the DM was quite interesting, and he never, at any time, seemed like he was bothered by my questions. In fact, just the opposite. He was overjoyed to talk about himself and his work. I stored this information for later use; maybe it would embolden me the next time I shied away from asking a stranger where she'd gotten her cute purse.

I saw firsthand how challenging the DM's job must be when a man wearing a ball gag and being whipped on one of the Xs started scream-

---

3   I learned that there are various types of boot play, but the most common is when a submissive licks, sucks, and shines the boots of his or her dom (or "dominant") partner. Sometimes the submissive is the one in boots with heels so high that it's impossible to walk in them, so she's at the mercy of her dom. This was my favorite fetish so far because it involved cool footwear.

ing. Was it a passionate-pleasure scream or a hey-that-really-hurts scream? Maybe the pain had made him forget his safe word.

I saw the DM sprint over and confer with the man briefly.

That had to be a difficult conversation.

> DM: Hey.
>
> FLOGGEE: [Through the ball gag] Heh.
>
> DM: How're you doing?
>
> FLOGGEE: Ar rokay.
>
> DM: All right. You're okay, then?
>
> FLOGGEE: Ar hine. Hodaly hine.
>
> DM: You're fine?
>
> FLOGGEE: Aherootly.

One of the prerequisites for the DM position: understanding ball-gag. I'd imagine most dentists are also fluent in it.

I finished chatting with the DM and felt prouder of myself than I guessed anyone else in the sex club was feeling that night.

I sauntered confidently back to Joe but was immediately sent off kilter again by a woman who was watching the *shibari* and getting fingered two feet away from us.

I shut my eyes hard for a second.

"You okay?" Joe asked. "You wanna go?"

"No," I said. "I'm good."

And I was good. It was just a lot. I love sex, but it was everywhere, and that got to be a bit much. This is the same reason I've never visited the Tillamook Cheese Factory.

I turned away from the *shibari* to get a quick break, but right behind us was a room with a naked couple engaging in full-blown sixty-nine. The room had a huge window, further enhancing the Sex Zoo feel of the place. I looked for the button to push to get info.

Humans aren't the only animals that engage in oral sex. Fellatio and cunnilingus are also enjoyed by Tibetan macaques, goats, brown bears, ground squirrels, and the particularly adventurous greater short-nosed fruit bat.[4] *Now please keep moving to your left, where you'll find an older couple on the sex swing who will make you think about your own mortality.*

That button didn't exist.

Joe and I went back to watching the *shibari* show and he started rubbing my lower back. He kissed me. I felt self-conscious about the PDA for a minute, but then I thought about the sixty-nine couple and the bar where a good twenty people were watching a man strategically poking his girlfriend with a magic wand while she dangled from the ceiling on ropes and giggled.

We were, by far, the least interesting thing in a fifty-foot radius.

As I watched the *shibari* performers behind the bar interacting with one another and with the patrons, I was struck by how collegial it all felt. At one point, the rigger for the two women slipped a little and they both bounced toward the mattress, then threw their heads back in giddy laughter as they righted themselves. These people seemed

---

4   This information is actually true. At least according to the "Animal Sexual Behaviour" Wikipedia page. I'm going to believe it, because the world is a more interesting place for me if I do.

to have real affection for one another, and even though they were all naked and being undeniably sexual, it didn't feel lascivious. It felt like they all had this hobby they loved and practiced a lot, and they were excited to be able to show it to people. It just so happened that some of them were having orgasms as they did it. It was sweet in the way that only Japanese rope torture can be sweet, you know?

This feeling may have been limited to fetish night; I didn't have anything to compare it to.

If Joe and I wanted to continue making out, we could choose our level of exhibitionism. We could, like the sixty-niners, grab a bed in a room with a giant window so everyone in the club could marvel at our skill, or we could duck into a sex-swing room with no door, or we could use one of the rooms with no windows and a door you could actually close and have some privacy. (The beds in those rooms had thick plastic mattress protectors that made the mattresses look like they were wrapped in body bags.) Or we could use the couples' room downstairs, which we hadn't explored yet.

I decided I wanted to see more of the first floor. That's where the actual bar and the infamous buffet was. We got a cocktail and decided to explore the couples' room.

We stepped into the large, cavelike room, which was decorated in a Japanese/late-model-Ikea-style with low light and lots of battery-operated fake candles flickering on all the exposed skin. There were eight futons, all evenly spaced about five feet apart, and each was sectioned off by a "curtain" of sheer fabric. On top of every futon was a sheet, a towel, and two condoms.

I'd expected all the beds to be filled with bodies engaged in new and innovative sex acts that would leave me feeling unimaginative, but it turned out people didn't necessarily go into the couples' room to have sex.

Sure, there was a couple in the first bed having sex. But the second bed was occupied by a fully clothed couple, each one sullenly sipping a drink; they looked like they'd run out of things to say. On the third bed, there were two couples—one fully clothed, one clearly postcoital—and the four of them were chatting. I heard one of them mention the final shootout on *Breaking Bad*.

Joe pointed out a bed in the corner next to another bed with five fully clothed people on it. They were chatting too.

Why aren't these people in a coffee shop? I thought.

Joe indicated we should sit down.

We covered the futon with the sheet and sat down. Then I grabbed another two sheets from a shelf of clean linens and covered that sheet with those because I figured there was no way one thin sheet could possibly be enough to protect us from the layers of smut residue in a club with Ron Jeremy's name on it. Then I wondered how many times the staff washed the sheets. Then I wished I'd brought a sheet of my own. Then I let the sheet thing go.

We talked for a bit as I peered through the gauzy curtains at the other couples and wondered what had brought them here. Were they exhibitionists? Swingers? Trying to spice up their marriages? I looked around and thought, *God, I have no idea what would have to happen in my relationship to get me to end up on a bed in the couples' room of a sex club.*

Then I realized that I was currently on a bed in the couples' room of a sex club, so clearly I had some idea.

Joe put his hand on my knee.

"How're you doing?" he asked. "Is this weird?"

It was nice that he kept checking in with me. How *was* I doing?

I was far more relaxed than I'd been when we walked into the club. I'd seen everything they had to offer that night, and while I'd never seen live sex acts before, I was amazed at how quickly it got boring. Maybe it was just the sheer number of them, but it definitely turned into a "you've seen one penis going into a vagina, you've seen them all" situation.

"Are you kidding?" I asked. "Of course this is weird. Don't you think this is weird?"

He looked around, running his hand softly along my back as he always did.

"Yup," he said. "Definitely. You wanna make out?"

"Seems like we should," I said. "Those guys are already way ahead of us."

I indicated a couple across the room who had come in after us but were already naked.

"Wait...do you want to have sex?" he asked.

"I don't know," I said. "I'm not sure."

"Well, definitely let me know when you know," he said.

He kissed me and I kissed him back. He put his arms around me, and we began kissing with purpose.

I started doing the emotional math.

Do I want to have sex with him tonight?

Absolutely.

Will I ever be in a sex club again?

Not likely.

Should I pull a "when in Rome" as long as I'm here?

I don't think most people in Rome would have sex in public at this point, so don't kid yourself by saying you're doing what the Romans do.

I don't know... I think I might regret it if I don't. It's like going to Disneyland and skipping Space Mountain, or going to the Louvre and running off to the Jamba Juice in the food court before you get to the Mona Lisa.

Is there a Jamba Juice at the Louvre?

It just seems like if you're going to go to a sex club, go to a sex club.

That's an excellent point.

Also, look around. Not a single person here is paying attention or gives a shit.

That one sort of clinched it for me. I undid his belt.

He seemed pleased.

Because we were in a public place, there was no way in hell I was going to get undressed. Because I'll have sex in front of total strangers, but God forbid I show my midriff.

I did my best to concentrate on Joe, but there was a group of people on the bed next to us talking about whether J. J. Abrams was going to ruin the Star Wars franchise. Also, there's a reason no one over thirty ever has sex on a futon: it's like fucking on a boulder with a slipcover.

Joe asked me some sexy questions while we were in the middle of it all. It was just your standard "Is that big enough for you?" and "You like that?" kind of thing, but I felt a little funny answering in front of everyone. They were kinda personal questions.

I answered very quietly.

I laughed a little when it was over and I was standing at the side of the futon getting my clothes and self back to normal again.

"What?" Joe asked, buttoning his shirt and looking for his shoe.

"Nothing," I said. "It's just a little odd to have sex in a room next to people casually discussing whether the auteur theory applies to sci-fi directors."

"Do you think it does?" he asked.

"Fuck yeah, it does," I replied. "I almost stopped you so I could say so."

As I sat on the futon putting on my shoes and chatting with Joe about the ridiculous thing we'd just done, I realized that this was the end of the line for me, sexual-experimentation-wise.

It was clear from my experience with Jeremy, and at Joe's house, and now this that sex simply wasn't an area where I needed to test my boundaries, because I might not have any.

I'd taken a foray into nontraditional relationships and it had been strange and illuminating, but it wasn't what I wanted. I'd been brain-washed by romantic comedies, and being someone's second was never the happy ending. (Although someone should make *When Harry Met Sally and Sally's Open-Minded Friend Who Works as a Cheesemonger at Whole Foods* for the poly age.)

If I really thought about it, this whole year was supposed to be about me becoming infinitesimally braver, not buying into my fears. And dating polyamorous people had always been a self-defensive act, meant to protect me from getting too emotionally involved and risking heartache. It was as if I was specifically seeking out people with whom I had nothing in common so I couldn't possibly fall in love with them.

And I wanted to fall in love.

I wanted those hours-long conversations where your whole body buzzes from the connection. I wanted unfettered, uncluttered access to someone who loved me with his whole heart because he hadn't given pieces of it to someone else. Someone who could choose to have anyone's back in the world but chose to have mine and mine alone. Back fat and all.

Thankfully, Joe and Jeremy had helped with my quest to find love by showing me what to look for in a sexual partner: sensual, sweet, intimate affection and filthy, no-holds-barred sexual bullying.

Finding both of those in one person might be a challenge.

Even though I'd decided that my big sexual-experimentation days were over, I still had to finish my evening with Joe.

Notably, we hadn't tried the buffet yet.

You may be asking, "Why the eff is there a buffet at a sex club?"

The answer is boring. According to Oregon Liquor Control Commission law, any bar serving alcohol must also serve "two different substantial food items."

Enter Build-Your-Own-Burrito Night[5] at Sesso.

The food looked fine, though out of place—less like bar food and more like what might be served at your aunt's fourth wedding at the local Elks Lodge. There were chafing dishes with Sternos, bowls sparsely filled with burrito ingredients, and disposable plates and utensils on a long table covered in a white tablecloth. I'd been expecting a sneeze guard at about crotch height, but I assume the NO NUDITY sign precluded the need for it.

At the buffet, we encountered what was by far the most disturbing part of the night.

They'd run out of tortillas.

---

5   *Build-Your-Own-Burrito Night at the Sex Club* is the title of my next book, so don't even try to call dibs.

I went through so many emotions. First shock, then denial ("How can you run out of tortillas at a burrito bar? It's the only crucial burrito ingredient. I can put lettuce into a tortilla and it's a lettuce burrito. I could put my phone in a tortilla and it's a phone burrito. I could go on, but I won't. I'm too upset"), and then I just settled into anger and disappointment.

Joe and I still filled our plates and sat in what would've looked like a break room at JCPenney if it weren't for the woman at the next table whose breasts had mostly freed themselves from the prison of her bustier.

Eventually I recovered from the tortilla thing and pulled it together, and sitting with Joe and Bustier Lady eating canned refried beans was the most comfortable I'd been all night.

"So you've done this," Joe said. "What'd you think?"

"Of the sex or of all of it?" I asked, still a little mad at the refried beans for not being inside a tortilla.

"All of it," he said.

"It wasn't very sexy," I said. "It felt really...performative. A lot of energy sent outward instead of shared, I guess."

"Some people find that sexy," he replied.

"Do you?" I asked.

"A little," he said. "My wife wanted the membership."

"I don't know," I said. "I guess I like my intimacy to be more...intimate."

"You're so square," he said, grinning.

"I guess I am," I replied.

I know the concept of a sweet poly guy who has a sex-club membership might sound contradictory to some, but Joe was just that, and maybe even a little out of place in this world. A man who goes poly to make his wife fall more in love with him seems rare. And even though I'd decided poly guys weren't for me, for those who are interested in emotionally lighter fare, I'd recommend dating poly guys like Joe, for a few reasons:

First, if he's married, you can be sure at least one person finds him attractive and interesting enough to agree to attempt to live with him for the rest of her life. And if the aforementioned wife is still alive, he's probably not a serial killer, which, in the online-dating world, is a plus.

Secondly, they're pros at communication. They have to be in order to navigate all the complications polyamory presents, like setting the rules of their primary relationships, negotiating the emotional complexities of two to three to four different romantic entanglements, and organizing the borderline-nightmarish logistics of an orgy.

And third, if and when you need to end it (like I had to), it's less painful for everyone, because your ex-partner has a permanent backup person and can avoid the inevitable "no one will ever love me" stage of a breakup.

At two a.m., after we finished eating our burrito ingredients, Joe and I stepped out of the club and into the cool air. He held my hand on the way to my car and kissed me before I got in.

"Night, square," he said, kissing my hand.

I smiled and got in the car. He was right. In the world of *shibari*, ubiquitous porn, and dungeon monitors, I might have counted myself among the squares. But out here in the real world, I felt decidedly hexagonal.

An Hour with a Professional Cuddler:

Wherein I Learn Not to Hate Affirmations . . . As Much

There are things in my life that I didn't know how much I needed until I got them.

Power steering.

My first really good knife.

A tiny computer I can talk into that has games, a calendar, and constant incoming messages to distract me from the ever-present knowledge that I'm going to die alone.

Oh, and touch.

I've known since my first relationship that physical affection was important to me. My first boyfriend had this insanely thick, silky head of hair that I loved running my fingers through.

"You're petting me again," he'd say as he was trying to fall asleep, and I would slowly pull my hand away, embarrassed by my constant desire to show him affection.

It was one of those situations where you feel like a total asshole until years later when you realize the asshole was the person who made you feel like an asshole.

Joe and I stopped seeing each other a couple weeks after we visited Sesso because I had decided the poly thing, while admirable in the emotional juggling department, wasn't for me. It ended amicably. I know this because we still follow each other on Twitter (#amicable). But being with Joe, I'd been reminded of what a priority touch was for me.

So when the opportunity arose to visit Samantha Hess, I knew I had to at least consider it.

Samantha is a professional cuddler.

She offers cuddling sessions featuring nonsexual touch at one dollar per minute. Sessions run anywhere from fifteen minutes to five hours. She originally operated out of her home, but she got so busy that in 2015 she opened Cuddle Up to Me studios and hired three other cuddlers, each of whom trained with her for forty hours.

You may ask why someone would need training to cuddle. Cuddling seems pretty self-explanatory. The only complicated part is deciding which spoon you are, which can get dicey. Being the big spoon can feel needy or overbearing, while some little spoons spend entire relationships cuddling against their will because they weren't honest in the beginning about being anti-cuddling and now they're trapped in a web of lies and their lovers' arms.

But I digress.

Samantha's snuggling apprentices needed training because her clients could choose from sixty positions of Samantha's creation, each with its own purpose and level of difficulty. There's the Blooming Lotus, where both participants are seated, legs wrapped around each other. There's the Cloak, where the cuddler simply lies facedown on top of the cuddlee's back. And of course, the Tarantino, where the cuddlee lies against a pillow and the cuddler sits opposite him, her feet on his chest, in an homage to Quentin Tarantino's alleged[1] foot fetish. (This one's only done with clients who don't sexualize feet, but if they don't, I'm not sure why they would want it.)

Samantha's storefront (and a really good publicist) garnered the attention of media outlets across the country and around the world, including *People* magazine, *Anderson Cooper 360* on CNN, and *CBS This Morning*.

This attention set off a virtual tidal wave of snark, and I get it—it's such an easy thing to take shots at. As comic Hari Kondabolu said on *Live Wire!*, "You don't have to be famous for people to say mean things about you on the internet. You just have to be earnest." There's nothing more earnest than offering yourself up to provide physical comfort. Add the layer of doing it for money, and you've got yourself some primo material for countless jabs.

Samples of comments on the stories about Samantha include *Sixty bucks an hour and I'm supposed to keep my pants on? No, thanks; It's really alarming if you have no one to cuddle with for free;* and, simply, *This sounds pathetic.*

While I didn't feel strongly enough about Samantha's profession to say something terrible about her on the internet, when my column

---

1   Note to Quentin Tarantino's lawyers: I said *alleged*. I don't know if this is true or not, so don't come at me. I loved *Reservoir Dogs*.

editor forwarded me an e-mail from Samantha's publicist with the note *Are you interested in this?*, my initial response was a resounding "Fuck no."

It's not that I don't think people should be able to pay for a cuddle if they want to. They should. It's just that when I thought about how trapped I would feel cuddling with a stranger for an hour, my stomach dropped, my dread ball appeared, and my expression morphed into what I call the Grimace of Anticipatory Dread.

I get it a lot. It's not attractive.

I stared at the e-mail for a few minutes.

Goddamn it.

Samantha was a stranger. I'd just had a breakthrough with a stranger at Sesso. Talked to him for a good five to seven minutes and then walked away as if it were nothing. Like a normal person. What if cuddling with Samantha acted as exposure therapy for my stranger problem? If I could cuddle for an hour with a person I'd never met before, then walking up to someone at a bar would be easy.

I also reminded myself, for what seemed like the millionth time, that one of the goals of this project was to prove to myself that a little embarrassment or discomfort wouldn't kill me. Most of us have had one-night stands (sorry, Mormons), and this would be, theoretically, a lot less intimate than that. Probably. Or maybe not.

I could do this. In fact, maybe I could get some cuddling tips from her. The only cuddling rule I was aware of was the cardinal one: Farting while one is the little spoon is a relationship-ending move. I had a lot to learn.

Turned out, this was actually the perfect time for me to get some cuddles in, since I'd decided to slow my dating life down to a crawl. I didn't think I knew what I wanted, and even if I did, it didn't feel like it was out there.

I set up the appointment with Samantha.

On the day of my session, I started feeling some creeping anticipatory dread early in the afternoon. Nothing that rose to the level of a panic attack, but the under-the-surface kind of anxiety that puts you on edge and makes you check your purse for Ativan before you leave the house.

Samantha's storefront was on Lower Burnside in Southeast Portland. A window display featured copies of her books and T-shirts with the store's logo: a simple illustration of a red heart with a circle at the top and two crisscrossed lines across the middle, turning the heart into a person being hugged.

Based on first impressions, I didn't think this was my style.

I arrived at the same time as my editor, who had joined me to take pictures, which only served to increase my level of discomfort, especially since he had clearly made up his mind about Samantha ahead of time (he was firmly in the snark camp). He looked pretty much exactly how you'd picture an editor would—a rail-thin man with five o'clock shadow, a fedora, and strong sense of irony.

The interior looked like it might've been a gym in a past life. No-pile carpet, white walls. A curtain ran along one side of the main room near the back, and the furniture was sparse and mismatched, which I forgave since she'd just opened up. A woman in her twenties with short red hair welcomed me.

"Are you Courtenay?" she asked.

No? "Yup," I said.

"I'll get Samantha!" she said. She seemed nice. Didn't help.

As soon as I met Samantha, I understood the draw. A five-foot-three impish brunette, she had a reassuring smile and a sweet, kind energy that would've put me at ease if I hadn't come in, as my friend Stacey's dad used to say, "wound up tighter than a clam's ass."

"You don't look excited about this," she said, grinning.

"I wouldn't say that I am," I said. "This isn't really a thing that I'd...y'know, normally..."

"Do?" she said.

"Nope," I said.

"I get that a lot," she said. "We won't do anything you're not comfortable with, and we can stop at any time."

She sounded like my dentist.

The buzzing in my chest had been at threat level 6, and that took me to about a 7. I tried not to imagine what we were going to do because that made it worse.

Like all new clients, I was given a clipboard with a questionnaire to fill out, a map of my body so I could indicate where it wasn't okay to touch me, and a waiver that lay down the ground rules. Among them were these: I was not to interpret the session as sexual; there would be no kissing; and touching would be limited to areas that were not normally covered by a swimsuit. (*What if I usually wear one of those old-timey swimsuits? Then I could just leave, right? Because you could only touch my ankles, and that's not cuddly.*) Clients were expected to have showered, brushed their teeth, and put on only a minimal amount of perfume, if any.

I don't think the client before me had gotten the memo on that one, because the patchouli smell coming out of the Beach Room rivaled the back of a Vanagon at a Phish concert.

Once I filled out the questionnaire, Samantha and one of her cuddlers-in-training came back to the consultation area behind the curtain for the pre-interview.

Samantha interviewed all her clients prior to cuddling with them, and, amazingly, this has kept her from having to end a single cuddling session early due to sexual inappropriateness.

"How is that possible?" I asked.

"I've trained my intuition," she said. "After some interviews, I have had to let potential clients know that my service isn't for them."

She said this generally happens with people who ask a lot of detailed questions about what's appropriate and what's not, and eventually it becomes clear that what they're looking for is sexual touch.

> CLIENT: What about the butt?
> SAMANTHA: Nope.
> CLIENT: Right under the butt?
> SAMANTHA: No.
> CLIENT: The front butt?
> SAMANTHA: We're done here.

I was about to ask another question, but she answered it before I could.

"Everyone always asks if men get erections," she said. "And of course they do, but that doesn't end the session."

"So how do you deal with it?" I asked.

"I've gotten really good at redirection and positions where it's not an issue," she replied.

I asked her why she thought she was so good at telling who might give her trouble. She told me that she'd watched her mother being physically abused when she was growing up.

"I've learned to really pay attention to the world around me," she said. "Those minute little cues people give you, like whether someone can look you in the eye or if they do that slow cat blink or look away a lot."

She said she used this same intuition in other ways, like sensing people's level of comfort when they touched her, how they responded or didn't respond, where they tensed up.

"Every new interaction I have, I'm putting in my calculator and figuring out what makes the most sense for them."

I imagined being in a relationship with a person like Samantha. It would be like dating a need ATM, someone who always gave you exactly what you asked for, even when you didn't know you were asking for it. It would be a little eerie.

Her biggest question for me in the pre-interview was "What brings you here?"

I told her about my discomfort with talking to strangers, my exposure-therapy theory, and how dating Joe had made me curious about physical affection in general—why I thought I needed it more than others and what that said about me. Was I overly needy physically? Was I cloyingly affectionate to my partners?

I also wanted to ask her if there was a way to solve the issue of what to do with the bottom arm when you're the big spoon—it's always a problem for me. But I decided that could wait for later.

Samantha said she could tell, based on my story and the fact that

I was wearing my shoulders as earrings, that I was comfortable with affection but very uncomfortable with the idea of getting it from a stranger. She assured me that I was in good hands.

I still felt something very similar to dental dread, and I am terrified of the dentist.

She showed me the four rooms I had to choose from, each with a bed and a bedside table, as my editor snapped away. The Beach Room was covered in seashells with blue waves painted on the walls; the Cascadia Room had trees, mountains, and wildflowers painted by a local artist; the deep burgundy Zen Room had the studio logo and an infinity symbol on the wall; and the Space Room had dark walls, a lamp with a spinning shade that threw a rotating aurora borealis all over the place, and glow-in-the-dark stars on the ceiling. I chose that one because it seemed best suited for imagining myself anywhere but there if the experience turned out to be utterly miserable. (I always plan for this eventuality. If I went on an African safari with Ryan Gosling, I'd bring my iPad just in case the tigers were busy licking their balls, and Gosling was a snore-fest, both of which were quite possible. When you're that pretty, you don't need to be interesting.)

I took my shoes off and got on the bed. My physical and emotional discomfort levels were both at a solid 11. My forearms were tingling, which, as I've pointed out, generally happens at the outset of an anxiety attack. Samantha was saying something, but whatever it was couldn't break through the buzzing in my head. She sounded like a teacher on a *Peanuts* special.

"Wah-wah, wah-wah-wah-wah," she said. "Wah-wah?"

I was sweating profusely and I couldn't look at her. I also couldn't look at my editor, and I definitely couldn't look at the camera. It's difficult to tell where my discomfort level would've been if he hadn't been in the room taking pictures. If I was already at an eight, the camera might have raised me to, say, a billion.

We'd agreed that he'd get a few shots and then leave so Samantha and I could have a real session.

It didn't help that he clearly thought what Samantha was doing was ridiculous.

I'd written fourteen columns at this point, and being photographed while cuddling was by far the most uncomfortable I'd been. And I'd just had sex in public.

Cuddling is already a vulnerable act. Receiving affection can make you feel vulnerable because people are often seen as weak for needing it. Offering affection makes you feel even more vulnerable due to the possibility of being rebuffed. Now imagine yourself in either of those positions but with a stranger. Being photographed. For the internet.

Discomfort level had now decreased to a 10 but only because I was lying down.

I love lying down.

Samantha asked me to sit up so we could attempt the first position, the Motorcycle. In this position, she sat behind me with her legs and arms wrapped around me, her head on my left shoulder. If she had been someone I knew, it probably would've felt lovely, but she was unfamiliar to me, so it felt...incongruous. Like your bank teller suddenly stroking your cheek. Also, because someone was photographing us, my brain was busy saying, *Camera! There's a camera right there. Where is it in relation to my chin(s)? Do my thighs look huge in this position? Is there any position in which my thighs don't look huge? Maybe if the camera were mounted in Skylab. The internet is going to eat me alive.*

I imagined the posts.

Of course she went to a professional cuddler. Who would ever touch her? Sad.

Eat a fucking salad. Jesus.

That may sound hyperbolic to you, but the internet is a cesspool.

I've gotten my share of abusive comments in the past, but the one I remember most was from seven years ago. My friend Shelley McLendon and I had mounted a ridiculous staged parody of the Patrick Swayze film *Road House.* We'd gotten a series of great reviews from our local weeklies, none of which I remember. But I do remember this comment on one of the reviews: *Wow. It'll be great to actually see Courtenay Hameister being funny in something. Is she playing the road or the house?*

I thought it must've been someone I knew, because who would be so cruel to a stranger who hadn't bitch-slapped one of his family members? And why did I remember nothing from the good comments but every single word of the bad one?

I've heard this phenomenon was once useful, that back when humans were hairier and less neurotic, their brains were trained to take special note of bad things, like Gork getting eaten by a saber-toothed tiger, so that they themselves could avoid becoming lunch. *Saber-toothed tiger = bad. I'll just replay that bloody scene a few times so you'll remember that,* said the prehistoric brain. (*Dear Evolution: Please stop working against us. It's getting old.*)

I know most people don't experience fear when being photographed, but when you've struggled with body issues your whole life, a camera might as well be a saber-toothed tiger. One that waits to bite you until you're tagged on Facebook or someone asks if you're currently portraying a building.

I tried to ignore the tiger and just be present/live in the moment/ feel my feelings as Samantha tried another position, this one called the Eiffel Tower, wherein we lay face to face, legs intertwined, each with one arm beneath a pillow, clasping each other's hands.

I had to agree with my editor on this one. It was ridiculous.

I could feel my face flush as the mortification of direct extended eye contact set in. People look at technology more than they look at one another these days, so direct eye contact feels almost... aggressive. Also, people don't just lie in bed staring at each other unless they're in a Nicholas Sparks movie or a mouthwash commercial.

I tried to concentrate on other things, like the fact that she had incredibly soft hands and a kind face.

I realized that I was looking in her left eye. I switched to her right eye. Then I tried to look in both eyes and my eyes started to cross.

I realized I wasn't technically breathing.

The shutter clicked, ratcheting up my dread.

I took a breath so I wouldn't die.

My palms were sweating.

She had to feel that.

I wanted to apologize for my sweaty palms, but what if, by some miracle of nature, she had no ability to sense wetness or dryness in her extremities, in which case I would just be calling attention to it without needing to?

I'm not sure exactly how long the eye contact lasted, but it felt like approximately one to two months.

Thankfully, Samantha started shifting to a new position, the Honeymoon. In this cuddle, I was on my back and Samantha lay in the crook of my left arm, her head resting on my chest and her arm around my waist. This felt unnatural. As a woman, I'm normally the one in the crook with a protective arm around my shoulder.

Even so, it was such a relief to be out of the eye-contact situation that I think the shift actually calmed me down a little. But I still had no idea how any of it would've felt without the fucking camera there.

Finally, I heard the comforting beep of a camera being shut off, and my editor said his good-byes. Now I could really see what this experience was like.

When the door closed, Samantha asked if I wanted to move into a different position. I'd thought I would want to, but I didn't.

I just wanted some time to breathe and see if it was at all possible to relax into this. I took a series of deep breaths and expanded my diaphragm to tell my parasympathetic nervous system that everything was copacetic.

Samantha's body felt like all the tension had flowed out of it. Her torso relaxed into me. She felt like a human weighted blanket.

She seemed utterly devoid of self-consciousness. I envied the shit out of that.

In the moments I managed to push my own self-consciousness aside, it actually felt nice to give comfort instead of receive it.

Prior to the appointment, I had expected that if I ever actually calmed down, all I'd want was to be taken care of—held, touched—and I'd specifically mentioned that I liked having someone run their fingers through my hair because what kind of asshole doesn't like that?

But it was interesting to discover that sometimes being taken care of means being allowed to offer affection to someone.

Samantha leads people through each session based on what she thinks they need; sometimes she tries multiple positions, sometimes the client knows exactly what she wants and it's just one or two positions for the whole hour.

Some clients want to give affection and comfort; some want to receive it. She says about 30 percent of her clients are women, and she finds they're pretty equally distributed into the giving and receiving categories. Once I finally relaxed, I liked both.

At one point I started to feel uncomfortable with the silence, so I asked her a question.

"So, do you sometimes find yourself training people to be better at intimacy?"

"Sure," she said, lifting her head to face me.

I couldn't shake how postcoital this conversation felt.

"I had one client who could only accept touch when he started, not give it," she said, turning her head and laying it on my chest again. "It took him about seven or eight months before he was giving touch, which was a great sign. When people want to give touch, it means they're in a good place in the world."

We lay there in silence for a little while.

"Why were you so uncomfortable with the camera in the room?" she asked.

"How did you know I was uncomfortable?"

"Your whole body was rigid," she said. "When he left, all your limbs went soft, like spaghetti."

I told her about my long history of hating my body. Of avoiding cameras or hiding behind furniture like Carnie Wilson in every Wilson Phillips video. Of saying terrible things to myself before other people could.

I told her about how I hadn't thought I was worthy of romantic love for over a decade as an adult because I was heavy. That I knew now how fat-phobic and downright tragic that was but that remnants of those feelings remained, like hateful little dust mites that I'd forgotten to sweep out of the attic of my brain.

She told me she'd struggled with body issues before she became a personal trainer but had found a way to accept herself when she learned about physiology and body mechanics. She realized that when she ate poorly, she gained weight, not because she deserved it but because of the math of calorie expenditure and metabolism. Apparently, when you don't see your body as a vessel that holds every mistake you've ever made, every shitty comment you've ever heard, and every Reese's Peanut Butter Cup you've shame-eaten in the bathroom, you can finally gain some perspective.

"Jesus," I said. "I can't even imagine what that would feel like."

"Why?" she asked.

"Because no matter what I weigh," I said, "I never stop feeling like a fat girl."

"What's wrong with being a fat girl?" she asked.

"Oh God...everything," I said. "It means I'm lazy, unhealthy, and have no self-control."

"Do you believe all that?" she asked.

"No," I said. "But yes. Those messages are everywhere when you're fat. Some people can escape them, but they seem like magicians to me."

I told her about losing all the weight after my gallbladder surgery and that I'd gained some of it back and was struggling again. I told her how much of my self-esteem came from whether I was eating healthily or unhealthily, and how my level of food intake defined whether I was a good or bad person. That I could save a toddler from a burning building, but if I was eating a cruller at the same time, the two acts would cancel each other out.

"Okay," she said, moving her head off my chest. "We're gonna do something. Sit up for me."

Oh, shit.

My stomach turned.

I didn't want to move.

But she was so *nice.*

I moved.

She had me turn slightly to the right and adopt the standard little-spoon position to her big spoon.

I'd never been spooned by a woman before. I'd recommend it. Women are soft and pillowlike.

She lay against my body, one arm wrapped around my waist, her left leg resting on my right leg, her limbs devoid of tension, like a marionette with no one holding the strings.

"We're going to do a few affirmations," she said.

This is the worst thing that's ever happened to me, and I drank a fly through a straw in sweet tea once.

"Okay," I said.

Silence. Maybe I'd gotten a reprieve. Maybe she'd fallen asleep.

"I am amazing," she said.

Oh Jesus.

I was hoping that wasn't the affirmation and that she was just telling me something she was super-proud of.

"I am amazing," she repeated.

"I'm... amazing," I said.

That wasn't so hard. I am sort of amazing. I'm here, aren't I? What non-amazing person would do this against her will? None.

"I'm enough," she said.

Ugh. Am I enough? I haven't filed my taxes for 2012 yet. I may be going to prison, so it feels like maybe...

"I'm..." she prompted.

"I'm enough," I said, then took a deep breath.

"I'm beautiful," she said.

I stopped breathing. I couldn't say it.

"I'm *beautiful*," she said again.

And I was crying. *A fucking affirmation is not making me cry.*

More than either of the others, this one caught in my throat. As much as I've always believed affirmations were full of shit, here was something they obviously could do: show me as clear as day what I believed and didn't believe about myself.

The tears from my left eye were now flowing into my right eye and then onto the pillow. Undeniable tears.

I could remember maybe three or four times in my life when I'd felt pretty, and this wasn't one of them. But even if I had felt pretty that day, I would never describe myself as being beautiful, as if it were a persistent state for me.

"I'm beautiful," she said.

She sounded like she believed it. But she *was* beautiful.

"I'm beautiful," I said, my voice breaking.

So. Humiliating.

Stop crying during your cuddle session. Stop it.

I had a trick to get myself to stop crying in public situations: I would imagine the first chest-burster scene from *Alien*. It'd worked for me when I had to read Shakespeare's Sonnet 116 at a friend's wedding.

She had me repeat the whole series of affirmations until I could say them without crying.

Finally, thanks to *Alien*, I could.

I can't say she made me believe them, but she made me believe that she believed them about me, which was almost as good.

When the moment was over, I wanted to say something to the effect of *We shall never speak of this again,* but that seemed inappropriate. I hoped that cuddler-client privilege was a thing.

As the session wound down, we lay there quietly and she ran her fingers through my hair. It wasn't exactly the same as having a lover or friend do it, but I have to say, it wasn't that different.

I have female friends who sometimes get massages because they need to be touched and know that if they don't, they might do something dumb, like sleep with a douchebag. Cuddling seems like a better choice for that purpose because it's far closer to the affection they're seeking than a massage.

I once read a study claiming that there's no discernible difference between the happiness you feel when you get exactly what you want, and the happiness you feel when you don't get what you want but convince yourself that what you did get was enough.

Cuddling felt like that to me.

You're getting affection, and whether or not you accept it is your choice.

I think part of the reason the affection felt so real had to do with Samantha. She was an anomaly in this age of irony and snark: a true optimist and an empath who believed that everyone deserves to be loved. I'm jaded as hell, and she convinced me. In the same way some people are more generous with money than others, I think there are people, like Samantha, who are perfectly willing to offer true affection—not guarded, not devoid of emotion—before someone has proven that he or she deserves it.

I think Joe was like this, which was why, even though our emotional connection wasn't strong, my experience with him was so powerful.

People who have access to physical affection all the time have no idea the emotional toll it takes on people who don't. Having spent so much of my adult life alone, I was hardly ever touched. Studies have shown that people who aren't touched are often lonelier, more anxious, and more likely to get sick than those who are. When you're never touched, it's only natural that you start believing that you don't deserve to be. The most tragic effect, though, is that those who haven't received affection often develop an anxious or avoidant attachment style, making it even less likely that they'll ever form relationships.

It doesn't take a genius, then, to determine why I might be more partial to physical affection than your average person. I'm like one of those kids whose parents were vegan so they got ice cream only once a year, on their birthdays, and then when they turned eighteen and left the house, they ate goddamned ice cream cake for dinner every night for two years.

These are my ice cream–cake years. And by that, I mean the rest of my life.

I understand why people are uncomfortable with what Samantha does, but in retrospect, I think the source of my own anxiety about seeing her was simple: I related to the people who needed her. I watched the world judging them and I felt judged too.

In the end, after all the initial strangeness wore off, I liked the session with Samantha because I like physical affection. I need it, even. And that doesn't make me needy or weak; it just makes me honest.

The question is, if I found myself alone for years at a time again, would I be willing to pay for touch? Maybe. At least with Samantha, I wouldn't have to get used to a whole new stranger.

The one problem with paying someone to touch you when you don't have that kind of touch in your life is that it has a marked poignancy; it's simultaneously exactly what you need and a reminder that you don't have it.

The fact that I hadn't been touched for the majority of my adult life had always been a source of shame to me, but even more shameful was why: I had come to believe that everyone hated my body as much as I did, so I simply wasn't open to it.

Maybe I was doing this whole thing backward—trying to find love before I figured out how to befriend my own body. Because you usually use your body in relationships, right? It's like half of the bodies in the relationship, I've heard.

Seeing Samantha also made me realize that I needed to change the dating portion of my adventure. I took down my online profile for a while until I could figure out how. I didn't know what I would or could do differently, but I was worn out from a series of short-term connections that were solely physical, and I was clearly in need of some comfort and true intimacy.

Which, to my surprise, I found.

Water Aerobics:

In Which I Learn How to Make Myself Feel (Relatively) Young and Attractive

Say what you will about Cathy Guisewite,[1] but she was right about trying on bathing suits. It's physically taxing and emotionally demoralizing and if the light bounces off your ass dimples just right, it can make you question every choice you've ever made.

Why didn't I keep playing soccer? you ask yourself while pinching your thigh fat. *If I had, I'd have lithe legs and look amazing in a pencil skirt and I never would've gotten laid off from that copywriter job. But I quit soccer like I quit everything that's the tiniest bit difficult. That's why I'm alone. I quit love too.*

---

1   If you're under thirty, Cathy Guisewite is the creator of *Cathy,* a comic that ran from 1976 to 2010 in which a professional lady waded through the complications of single life, ate too much chocolate, and said "Ack!" a lot. She tried on bathing suits inordinately often, especially for someone who claimed to hate doing it. Maybe it was a self-flagellation fetish. We'll never know.

"You okay in there?" the salesperson asks. "You need another size?"
Why are you even using the word size? *Do you hate me?*

That was me in December, after I slowed my dating roll for a while and took a mental-health break.

After not seeing a public pool in decades, I had water aerobics recommended to me by my doctor.

For the preceding year, I'd had some back trouble. Some days it would be fine, and some days I'd wake up and have to roll over onto my stomach, slide my legs off the side of my bed until they hit the ground, then push myself up to standing. It was very sexy in an "Estelle Getty on *Golden Girls*" kinda way.

All of this was due to what can only be described as the scourge of the cougar community: a Zumba[2] injury. It was bound to happen after a lifetime of never exercising and then five to six Zumba classes a week. (I took these classes during the health-panic months that followed my gallbladder surgery, during which I ate perfect low-fat meals and quite literally exercised my ass off.)

My previously unused spine was now being yanked around mercilessly for an hour a day, and it was confused and angry. At the L4 and L5 positions in my lower back, the disks whose job was to cushion the vertebrae decided it was all too much and tried to escape by partially squishing themselves out the back of my spinal column. This resulted in what's known as herniated disks, and they can irritate your nerves and cause excruciating pain all the way down your legs. Any person

---

2   For those of you who aren't Prius-owning women in their late thirties or early forties, Zumba is a fitness class that incorporates hip-hop, merengue, salsa, samba, mambo, and some martial-arts movements. It was one of my first OFW adventures. I hated it. Then I loved it.

who's hit forty and uses his or her back for things is probably familiar with them.

It was my pissed-off disks and the fact that I had gained back about twenty of the sixty-five pounds I'd lost and seemed to be continuing that trend[3] that led me to the dressing room at a great vintage-inspired swimsuit store called Popina in Northeast Portland.

I wanted to get back to a place where I felt good about, and in, my body. And because my back was a mess, my doctor thought the best exercise for me was a water aerobics class.

"You mean, like, in a pool?" I asked.

"That's where it generally happens, yes," she replied.

"Can't I just walk or something?" I said.

"You could, but at this point, walking for long distances might do more harm than good," she said. "You need to give your back a bit of a rest."

"Lying on the couch is resting," I said.

She smiled. "I know it sounds counterintuitive, but you have to exercise in order for it to get better," she said.

I shook my head.

Fucking pools.

I could've ignored her, but once again, life was throwing me an op-

---

3   Many women are comfortable dating while fat, and I salute them. There are tons of men who are attracted to heavier women; just do a search for *BBW* on a porn site and then revel in the wealth of thick ladies doing filthy things for money. (Hooray for equal-opportunity filth!) That being said, I was clearly not one of those women, and because dating already made me feel vulnerable, I wasn't willing to allow one more chink in my armor, since it already felt like a crumpled Diet Coke can.

portunity to do something that would fit nicely into the OFW Project if I let it. I'd done so many things I hated the idea of already, and once I'd done them, I hated them only a little. Maybe this would be the same.

At Popina, I struggled for half an hour with spandex and regret, and I left with the only thing that worked: a two-piece that covered my belly and had a grandma skirt to hide the tops of my thighs.

That's the suit I wore to the Aqua Fit class at my gym,[4] LA Fitness.

Aqua Fit is a class for people who have difficulty doing exercises that are jarring to the joints. Just picture a slo-mo aerobics class.

Sounds simple enough, right?

It would've been if I could've attended the class fully clothed and if it hadn't been in a freaking pool.

I'd passed the pool in my gym many times back when I used to go a lot, and I always wondered whose idea it was to have floor-to-ceiling glass windows that allow everyone to see in. This may be a form of motivation for people who are proud of their bodies, but it seems like a Shame Thunderdome for the rest of us.

I'd spent most of my adult life eating exactly what I wanted and exercising exactly as much as I wanted, which was only slightly more often than never. So all I had to do to trigger a shame spiral was reveal the result of that action and inaction in a public place. Actually, I didn't have to do anything to trigger a shame spiral. Just sitting often did it. Or waking up. It's a skill.

On the day of the first class, I decided to wear my bathing suit un-

---

4   If you've been through the doors of a gym one time in the past year, you get to call it "my gym," right?

der my clothes so I could just take off my skirt and sweatshirt and throw on my towel and no one in the locker room would see the body for which I would be mentally apologizing for the next hour.

When you're heavy and you attend a group fitness class, it's not totally out of the realm of possibility that your very presence is a cautionary tale for some attendees.

What a coincidence you're here, you imagine a skinny girl saying. *I'm here so I won't end up looking like you.*

I was able to walk right into LA Fitness because, despite all evidence to the contrary, I still had a membership there. I hadn't used it for over seven months, but it was important to me to have it there, waiting for me when I was ready. Also, I was apparently really angry at two hundred dollars and wanted it out of my bank account for no reason whatsoever.

When I got into the locker room, I pulled off my skirt and shirt and put on my towel in a very ungraceful thirty seconds, then walked down the hall toward the pool. As I approached the doorway, the smell of chlorine became stronger, as did my apprehension. I tried to imagine if there was any way for me to enter the room and drop my towel while simultaneously leaping into the pool at such a speed that it would be impossible for anyone to focus on any one part of my body. At the very least, my spider veins would be blurry.

Were those spider veins or a tattoo? a guy in the class would ask.

I don't know, another guy would respond. *She was moving too fast to tell. Our attempt to tread water in silent judgment has been thwarted.*

I was still forming my towel-ditching plan when I opened the door to the pool and everything changed.

The class wasn't filled with mean girls. It was filled with sexagenarians, septuagenarians, and octogenarians, all smiling at me encouragingly.

I felt almost all the tension in my body leave with my exhale.

I walked over to a hook on the wall, hung my towel up like a normal person, and stepped into the pool. I took a quick visual poll, and, yes, I was definitely the youngest person in the class by at least twenty years.

Of course the Aqua Fit class had senior citizens in it. It was for people who had back problems. And knee problems. People who were only marginally ambulatory. People like me. But miraculously, the class wasn't making me feel old.

Just a few weeks prior to the class, at a club where a friend's band was playing, the bouncer had laughed a little and waved me through when I tried to show my ID. As I walked through the club, desperately trying to spot my gray-templed friends among the young hipster crowd, I realized it was the first time I'd felt self-conscious about my advancing age in a social situation.

This was the opposite of that.

The Aqua Fit pool was the pool in *Cocoon* for me. Just stepping in made me magically appear young and vigorous. *Appear* being the operative term.

Our teacher, Molly, an effervescent woman in her late twenties with a swimmer's wide, powerful shoulders and tan, dimple-free legs, stood at the edge of the pool and demonstrated the moves. Which frankly look a little silly if you're not in water.

I moved to a spot in the shallow end. I admit that I was already judging Molly harshly for her Chinese-character tattoo because I was jealous of her leg muscles.

I'm sure it says something really great, I thought as I fought my inner judgmental bitch and the urge to find my phone and Google the character for "General Tso's chicken."

I should add that when I'm uncomfortable, I tend to get testy and lash out. Usually, the attack is directed at myself, but the people around me can also get some mental shrapnel.

We began with a lot of punching and kicking, some of it while standing up and some while floating horizontally and holding the edges of the pool. My doctor had told me that these classes could be good for increasing strength because there's quite a bit of resistance. But since it's resistance in the form of clear, blue refreshing water, it's about a million times more pleasant than an aerobics class on dry land. Those involve sweat and wheezing and complicated choreography and young, bright-eyed girls with their whole exercise lives ahead of them who jump higher than you ever could because they live on clouds of kale smoothies and completed to-do lists.

I was so relieved not to feel that pressure to perform. Yet.

For the first kicking session, I moved to the side of the pool next to an Asian woman with the face of a seventy-five-year-old and the body of a thirty-five-year-old. I wondered how one could still have taut arm skin at that age. It was extraordinary. She smiled and nodded at me as we both grabbed the edge of the pool. Molly blew her whistle to start the first fifteen-second kicking session. My back twinged a little as I kicked, but eventually the twinge went away and I started scissoring my legs as fast as I could. Which, it turned out, wasn't very fast.

That has to be fifteen seconds, I thought after five seconds.

I looked to my right, and my neighbor's legs were running like an Evinrude, water flying everywhere, while her face was serene and relaxed, like she was on a pool float holding a margarita. She turned to me and smiled, then turned back and kept going.

How dare she rub it in like that.

I was doing one-Mississippis and we were definitely past fifteen seconds, but Molly's whistle didn't go off. My muscles were starting to hum. Had she lost her whistle? Should I order one for her on Amazon? With Prime Now, it could get here in like twenty minutes.

Finally, she blew her whistle and we stopped to rest.

"That was good," my neighbor said. "Is this your first class?"

Ah, I get it. I see what you're doing.

"Yeah, how could you tell?" I asked.

"Oh, I've been coming to this class for a few years now," she said. "I just haven't seen you before."

Uh-huh. And you're so good now, is that what you're saying? What's next, "Float like a butterfly, sting like a bee"?

"Wow," I said. "That's a long time."

"It's all relative," she replied with a smile.

Was she talking about how fifteen seconds was really long for me but was super-short for her? Why was she so cruel?

"Okay! Now we're gonna go for thirty seconds!" Molly yelled.

Her whistle echoed off the tiles and the whoosh of twenty-four elder-legs kicking into gear immediately followed. I knew the Mississippis wouldn't help this time so I just braced for this set to feel like an hour. I slowed down my pace when my muscles started to ache and I looked down the line at my classmates, their legs flying in and out of the water at twice, maybe three times, my speed.

I couldn't believe I'd been lulled into a false sense of security by my ageism.

I was just as shitty in this exercise class as I'd been in every one I'd ever taken, but this one had the added humiliation of my classmates being approximately twenty years older than me and probably injured in some way.

Molly took us all the way up to a minute of kicking, which I horizontally hobbled through, then back down to fifteen seconds.

Exercises like this where I don't have a mini-TV in front of me are a real test of both my endurance and my attention span. I have trouble paying attention to stuff I *like* for longer than five minutes. This felt like water torture.

Just when I was grateful to finally be done with the kicking, we started in on jumping jacks, which I thought had fallen out of favor in the '80s with the advent of aerobicizing. They hadn't, apparently, but mine were still as stilted and unwieldy as they'd been in middle school.

Abe, a cranelike bald man with bright green eyes who looked to be about eighty and sounded like he was from Brooklyn, introduced himself to me while grabbing me a couple of floating barbells.

"You're doing good," he said with the same tone one might use when teaching an uncoordinated child how to perform neurosurgery.

"Don't patronize me, Abe," I said, only half kidding. Clearly they didn't get a lot of new students in this class, and they apparently saw me as a project.

"Everything takes time to get used to," he said.

Abe and I pushed the floating barbells underwater as Molly instructed us to, using the principle of buoyancy to benefit our pecs.

Then Molly had us walk and run the width of pool, still in the water, back and forth repeatedly. As we were passing each other, Abe introduced me to his friend Ron, who tipped an invisible hat to me.

I began to actually enjoy strolling in the pool with the cast of *Cocoon*, but as our speed increased, I noticed that the amount of water I displaced when I ran was far more than anyone else in the class did. This wasn't due to my youthful vigor; it had more to do with my mass.

I started to move more slowly so that the waves at the side of the pool didn't splash up as much.

I normally feel the impact of my size in tight spaces like airplane seats or skinny restaurant booths. It was disappointing to feel it in an Olympic-size pool.

As I slowed down my walk to try to take up less pool space, I remembered a conversation I'd had with my friend Lidia, an extraordinary author and teacher who also happened to be an avid swimmer.

I'd told her I'd gained weight after my back injury and that that made me feel vulnerable on dates and even more when I performed the bits I still participated in on *Live Wire!;* I imagined people who had heard me on the radio would be disappointed to see me in person.

Lidia said that she'd gained weight in the past few years too.

"It bothered me for a while," she said. "But now I have a new middle-aged-lady mantra with regard to my current body: I'm exactly as big as I need to be to write the kinds of books that I do."

I loved that sentiment at the time—it sounded so warm and accepting, so...evolved.

Was that why I couldn't stop eating Red Robin's bottomless fries?[5] Was I just trying to make my body big enough for my voice?

It didn't feel that way. It felt like food was a replacement for the romantic love I wasn't getting because I'd eaten too much food and therefore couldn't imagine finding romantic love.

Of course, food wasn't *just* that. Food was also comfort and pleasure and warmth and fullness and safety and actual sustenance and entertainment and sweetness and a delicious defense against absolutely everything that scared me or filled me with regret. Food was an emotional moat. Filled with gravy.

But what if food wasn't a defense and my body wasn't too big? What if I tried on the idea that my body needed to be this size to hold all the important things I had to say?

Act as if, I thought.

That's an old line that I first encountered while studying acting in college, but it's one that's been repeated by therapists over the years. What if you were brave enough? What if you were a person who could tell someone he hurt you, or ask for a raise, or get on a plane without having a panic attack? Do you know a person who can do that thing you cannot do? Imagine you're her. Now imagine doing the thing.

What if I just acted as if I were as evolved as Lidia at her best moments? What would that look like? What would it feel like? Would I be embarrassed by the ripples I was making or proud of them? Or would I not give a shit either way?

---

5   I'm usually a giant anti-chain snob, but Red Robin's steak fries dipped in ranch dressing made me fall in love with the strip mall by the airport, and I don't care who knows it. Except that I sort of do, but now the truth is out there so I just have to live with it.

That's when I started to experiment. I started walking faster and punching my arms more vigorously. I started making larger ripples with each pass, pushing my ample body through the water as bigger and bigger waves flowed over the side of the pool.

Turns out it's way more fun to try to displace water than try to contain it.

And it was also more fun to actually inhabit my body instead of trying to pretend I was in a different one.

I was actually enjoying myself. In a pool.

I make waves, motherfuckers! I thought. *I'm a tsunami. Deal with it.*

My version of Lidia, it turned out, was very aggro.

It felt amazing to be her for even a few minutes. To let go of my shame and imagine that my size had no other meaning or purpose but to send me more forcefully through the world.

I don't think anyone else in the class was having a water-related epiphany, so when Molly blew her whistle, I had a moment of self-consciousness, worried that the regular attendees were reconsidering their decision to welcome the middle-aged whippersnapper into the fold.

They seemed fine. It's good that people can't see your thoughts.

I stood in place as I was told, winded from the exertion but invigorated. I imagined this was what people who actually liked exercise felt.

Molly ended the class with us standing tall and running our hands through the water, one after the other, in a sweeping Mr. Miyagi motion.

Watching my hands move slowly under the surface and seeing the small waves they made became meditative, like underwater tai chi.

It seems smart to start the day concentrating on clear proof of the force you exert on the world. There's also something poetic about preparing for the day by running through water. Once you've spent an hour pushing through something with eight hundred times the pressure of air, moving through actual air is a cinch.

Bring it, world. I worked out with senior citizens this morning.

After Molly dismissed us, I walked over to the pool steps with my classmates, allowing most of them to get out before me.

"You did good," said Abe, patting my shoulder.

"Thanks," I said. "So did you."

He dismissed me with a wave. "I always do good. I'm a natural athlete," he said.

Ron rolled his eyes and got out of the pool.

"We gonna see you next week?" he asked.

"You might," I said, thinking it might actually be true.

As soon as I stepped out of the pool, I became me again, obsessed with who was walking behind me and how much the size of my ass bothered them. Even so, it didn't erase the glimpse I'd gotten of who I could be.

With a shit-ton of therapy.

After my small win in the pool, I took a quick shower and then, due to my inexperience with gym showering, attempted to put on a sports bra without properly drying myself. I spent two frighteningly squirmy minutes with my arms locked over my head in a stretchy black Lycra prison. At one point, I actually became claustrophobic enough that I almost asked a stranger for help.

When that seemed too humiliating, I spent a few seconds thinking, *Okay. I guess this is where I live now.*

Eventually, I managed to corral my boobs, but it wasn't lost on me that after bravely conquering aqua aerobics, I had almost been beaten by a piece of clothing whose whole job was to support me.

So I left the gym feeling less victorious than I'd felt in class, but still. It was enough that I'd finally had a life-affirming moment in a pool.

It was about time.

Adventures in Dating III:

Winter Is Coming

After my experience with polyamory and the tortilla debacle at the sex club that I still really hadn't recovered from, I'd backed away from the online-dating hamster wheel considerably. I thought it was time to either get serious about compatibility or quit altogether, both of which were equally possible given my mood at that point.

OkCupid was still the catalyst for the majority of my dates. I continued my quest, though at a more leisurely pace, sifting through thousands of pictures of men standing on mountains in hiking gear. Or skiing gear. Or "Holy shit is that Everest base camp?" gear.

I wasn't the outdoorsy type and listed *hiking avoidance* as a hobby in my profile so in the Northwest, I was an outlier.

Even so, I had managed to find over twenty Portlanders so far who (a) didn't make me start a fire using two rocks to test my camping mettle; (b) didn't have gluten allergies; and (c) didn't already know me. (Portland is a small town, so you will see friends and acquaintances on dating sites. The plus side is that it's similar to seeing them in a brothel or at an Arby's—the mutual mortification will keep your secret safe forever.)

I decided that if a person's profile or message didn't make me laugh, he wasn't in consideration.

That tactic got me a date with Taken Guy—another handsome, bearded forty-something who worked at Dark Horse Comics and let me know immediately after our date that he'd just started seeing someone else exclusively. There was also Crying-on-the-Inside Guy (a stand-up comic who teared up when talking about his ex-girlfriend). And then, in late October, my favorite suitor to date, Delayed-Text-Response Guy.

First Date #25, Late October: Delayed-Text-Response Guy

He was dorkily funny, darkly handsome, and bald in that Stanley Tucci–esque sense where it just fits and you can't imagine him any other way. He was an architect who spent a lot of time on construction sites, and his T-shirts always had what my friend Mimi used to call the "cool hang." That's where the shirt looks like it'd been washed a thousand times so it billows slightly at the bottom from stretch and wear. I've always had a strange affinity for guys who could achieve the cool hang, but maybe that's because I could never pull off a T-shirt. I always look like a roadie for a metal band.[1]

---

1   There is nothing wrong with being a roadie for a metal band. I just am not one.

On our first date, aside from the fact that I almost spilled my entire girlie cocktail when I stood up to greet him, we seemed to have fantastic chemistry. There were no cringe-filled conversational lags, neither of us talked more than the other, and we laughed easily at each other's borderline-TMI personal stories.

His only flaw, I noticed in the first week, was that he never took less than two hours to respond to a text and would sometimes take a couple of days. His replies always seemed interested and engaged, so I tried not to think about it.

Also, the fact that he was funny, even just a little bit, made me very hopeful. More hopeful than I'd been in a while, actually. Since I had started this dating binge months earlier, I'd found that humor was the rarest trait to come across. Out of the hundreds of profiles I read, probably seven made me laugh. And one of those seven was cribbed directly from a Best of Craigslist post from five years prior.[2]

I started thinking that since *funny* is at the top of virtually every straight woman's must-have list, Portland had simply run out of funny men, and we would have to start importing them from Canada.

So after Delayed-Text-Response Guy made me laugh on our first date, I was thrilled when he asked me on a second. We went to a bar in Southeast Portland where we sat at a long picnic table on the back

---

2 That guy was a real charmer—it took him only three texts to send me a dick pic. Once I discovered what he'd done (plagiarized Craigslist) and called him on it, he desperately tried to prove he wasn't a bad guy by sending me a picture of his four-year-old daughter, which only added to the creep factor, since it came right after the dick pic. I told him that the act of procreating did not automatically make one a good person. I love technology, but sometimes I miss the ability to slam down a phone receiver on someone who desperately deserves it.

patio surrounded by Edison-bulb string lights and tatted-up millennials who made us feel old simply by existing and being of drinking age.

"They all look like my daughter," he said.

"That's not helping," I said.

We swapped a lot of stories that night. He even told me about when he'd lost his virginity.

"Her parents were out of town so we had the whole house to ourselves for a weekend," he said.

"That's amazing!" I said. "You were so lucky."

"Well, yeah," he said. "It felt that way. But then she lost a tampon in her body somewhere and it started to feel more nightmarish than idyllic."

"'Somewhere'?" I asked.

"Well, I knew where it was," he said. "I just didn't want to think about it."

"Did you go spelunking for it?" I asked.

"I did," he said. "The weekend turned out to be instructive in a different way than I'd hoped."

"You probably never thought it was possible to see too much vagina."

"Absolutely," he said. "Turned out it was."

Even after that nonsexy sex talk, I decided to go home with him that night. It was our second date.

Here's why that might have been a mistake: There's an unspoken agreement among the majority of daters, and that's that the *third* date is the sex date.

I have no idea how it happened—I must have missed the summit where the decision was made—but it's a thing now.

For men, unspoken sex rules are not really an issue because they can fuck whoever they want whenever they want and however many times they want, and as long as their bodies don't become covered in syphilitic sores, there's not a lot of judgment.

But women need to be aware of things like the Third-Date-Sex Rule, because for some men, a woman's decision to sleep with him or not flips a switch in his mind, thus:

Sex on the first date = whore

Sex on the second date = whore

Sex on the third date = marriage material!

Some strange magic apparently happens to women in the time between the second and third date that sucks all the whore blood from our bodies and reanimates us with the blood of Donna Reed.

Of course I don't want to be with a man who thinks this way, but the problem is, some men think this way but don't realize it. Their penises and degrees in postfeminist lit think women should be able to do whatever they want with their bodies, but some dark part of their brains that they never visit is playing episodes of *Father Knows Best* on a loop and wagging a finger at hussies.

Since I'm terrible at game-playing and think the Third-Date-Sex Rule is garbage and that the people who subscribe to it are garbage people, I don't generally obey it, and I definitely didn't with Delayed-Text-Response Guy.

Did I sleep with him too soon for him to consider me serious dating material? I asked myself that question as his text-response time got longer and longer, and he became cool and distant on our third date. As we sat in his living room, he stared past me as we talked and looked down at his phone a few too many times.

Oh, is that another woman you're taking too long to respond to? Do you need me to give you a minute so you can not text her?

After that date, I was pretty sure he was attempting to ghost me, but I was so sure we were perfect for each other that I kept texting him every couple of weeks to see if he might want to go out. He would respond sporadically and claimed he was still interested when I flat-out asked him about it over text. (If nothing else, this dating thing had made me exceptionally good at using digital media to ask uncomfortable questions.)

It was completely bizarre that I continued pursuing him despite his obvious ambivalence. For a person with my paralyzing fear of rejection, this was akin to someone pursuing a hungry bear while decked out in Lady Gaga's raw-meat dress.

The only way I can explain it is that I really liked him, and that haze of affection made me blind to his not really liking me.[3]

But then I got a text from him with a vague excuse for why he had to cancel our fourth date, and for whatever reason, the fog lifted and I knew. I knew I was being passively broken up with via text by another guy I wasn't really dating. I was in the car driving home and when Siri read the text to me, I had to pull over because I was tearing up. (Side note for coders: Would it be so hard to engineer Siri to comfort users immediately following a breakup text? Just something simple like "I never thought he was tall enough for you" or "Do you want me to hack into his bank account and suck out the hundred dollars you paid for the morning-after pill?" You're the ones

---

3   You can scoff, but I've actually seen long-term marriages that follow this
     structure exactly.

who created this easy-breakup technology, so it's the only responsible thing to do.)[4]

Yes, crying because a guy you've had three dates with isn't interested in you seems a little over-the-top, but at that point, I was so tired. He'd been first date #25 and one of only about three men over the course of the year that I thought there might be a future with. But that estimation was clearly based on sparks that only I saw. And it's embarrassing, but I'd pictured myself with him. I pictured him coming to parties with me and putting his hand in the small of my back as we weaved through the crowd. I pictured us going to comedy shows and laughing at all the same jokes. I pictured my friends being impressed by the cool hang when I took him to barbecues. So when he pushed me aside, I wasn't just mourning three (mostly) good dates, I was mourning the future I'd prematurely imagined with him and, if I'm honest, the corgi I envisioned us adopting. (His name was General Alfred P. Biscuits, and his ears were as tall as a roll of Ritz crackers.)

When things start off so well and end so quickly, I'm always torn about whether I want to know the reason. Of course, on the one hand, it's way more pleasant not to know what it was about you they disliked enough to disappear on you, but on the other hand, a quick note of explanation could put an end to the obsessing over *why*. No one wants to hear, "I just don't think the spark is there," or "I would've married you if you'd just waited one more date to sleep with me, *whore*," but I spent a good couple of weeks ruminating on what

---

4   Fun fact: Text messaging was first conceived of by Finnish engineer Matti Makkonen, and the first text message was sent on December 3, 1992. The text was from Matt to his girlfriend and it said, *We need to talk.*

it might have been, and I could've used that time to ruminate about other important things, like how and when I was going to die or suddenly develop schizophrenia or that version of catatonia where you can't move or speak but you're aware of everything.

In November, because Delayed-Text-Response Guy had been the straw that broke my already-emotionally-fragile camel's back, I didn't actively try to date anymore.

I deactivated my OkCupid profile for the third time in a year, and I felt relieved.

I understood the appeal of having a whole catalog of prospects at your fingertips to choose from, but after a year of it, I just wasn't sure it was that effective. Or fulfilling. Or worth risking herpes.

I was also concerned about how my psyche had been affected by the illusion of plenty that online dating creates.

Let's be honest: The idea of a person is almost always better than the reality. When you go on a date with someone you met online, you carry with you the idea of literally thousands of people waiting on a website you can access at any time. So you're a lot less likely to give the person in front of you the chance he deserves, because how can he compare to all those possibly perfect people?

I wondered if this might have long-term effects.

If I ever did get into a relationship, wouldn't I keep the idea that I could shop online for another person in the back of my mind? So the moment I got bored or he got an unflattering haircut, maybe my impulse would be to hop back into the digital dating pool.

Part of what keeps a person in a relationship is that inner voice saying there's no one else out there. Online-dating sites are immediate, constant proof that that voice is full of shit. I'm not saying the lack of perceived alternatives is a good reason to stay in a relationship, but I think too many perceived alternatives can lead to people jumping ship when the ship they're in is quite sound, it just has a couple of totally fixable dents in the hull.

All of this is to say that I felt really good about my decision to take down my online profile. Deleting dating apps freed up a ton of time and mental space and I was getting a lot more done. I was writing more and spending more time drinking with my friends, which I'd missed terribly.

And, shockingly, I went on a couple of dates (#26 and #27) that were not arranged by an algorithm. Nothing of note, though, aside from a delicious piece of prime rib.

But once Thanksgiving was over, I was reminded again of the shitshow that being single in December is. My birthday. Christmas. New Year's fucking Eve, which is a million times worse than Valentine's Day because the whole world is kissing at the exact same time you're hiding in the bathroom looking at your phone and trying to avoid thinking about the whole world kissing. I've spent many first moments of new years in bathrooms.

I reactivated my OkCupid account the second week of December.

That's when I started getting messages from an engineer who liked cars.

First Date #28, December 26

So what if it was only half the field hockey team? Still too much? How about just one really unattractive midfielder as long as I promise never to do it again?

That was the first line of his message to me. I'd said in my profile that I thought humor was really important and that if a guy was funny, I'd forgive a lot. *Not sleeping with a whole field hockey team,* I'd said, *but a lot.*

Smart move, #28. He was letting me know that he'd actually read my profile (you'd be amazed how many don't), and the concept that indiscretions didn't count if the person one cheated with was unattractive was a real conversation-starter.

> HUSBAND: I've had an affair.
> WIFE: How could you?
> HUSBAND: No, no—it's fine! She looks like a less attractive Benedict Cumberbatch.
> WIFE: Oh. Sorry. My bad. More coffee?

We corresponded for four days, which was a little long for me. Now that I was an experienced online dater, I was more in the "meet in person before you form an attachment" camp. I was amazed at the number of fiery conversations I'd had online that froze over the moment they were exposed to real-world air and lack of physical magnetism.

And #28 had physical magnetism. His profile said he was six five (which I took with a grain of salt but was nice to imagine). He had close-shorn silver hair, a long, Roman nose, and deep-set blue-gray eyes. He looked a lot like Roger Sterling from *Mad Men,* which immediately made me imagine our Roger and Joan Halloween costumes.

But I was getting ahead of myself, as usual.

After about six notes back and forth, he asked me on a date. This was on December twentieth, so there wasn't a lot of open space in anyone's schedule. My birthday was Christmas Eve and my family loses their ever-loving minds at Christmas, so obviously that was out.

He suggested the twenty-sixth, which fell on a Friday, and I agreed. We met at a whiskey bar across from the theater where we recorded *Live Wire!*

Turned out he *was* six five, long and lanky, and therefore very possibly not a liar about other things. And unlike most of the dates I'd been on during the year, he'd actually dressed up to see me in a long-sleeved blue dress shirt and flat-fronted gray pants. He looked dapper as fuck.

We sat at the bar facing each other and talked for four hours.

He was soft-spoken and ridiculously smart, able to call up arcane facts about whatever subject we happened to be discussing with an unassuming ease.

He was a very recently separated engineer who ran a computer-chip factory in Hillsboro, a suburb of Portland. He had two kids, a nineteen-year-old daughter and a seventeen-year-old son who was autistic. His daughter was in college in Florida and his son lived with him.

I hadn't imagined dating a father who still had a kid at home, but after the year I'd had, I was willing to keep an open mind. When I looked back on my year, I realized it was kind of important that he was too. It had been an eventful year, during which I'd tried my darnedest to make up for my sexless twenties. In that sense, at least, it had been a glorious success.

I had my first and second (!) one-night stands, which shocked me at the time since they seemed so out of character for me, but in retrospect I saw them as a dating rite of passage.[5]

I dated three polyamorous men.

I went to a sex club and sampled more than the buffet.

I doubled my overall sex number, which took me from below average (more than a nun, less than a bi-curious girl on *rumspringa*) to above average (more than your mom, less than Axl Rose at Burning Man), which felt like a huge accomplishment to me.[6] I'd always been embarrassed by my late start, and while I'm sure my mother would never see it this way, I'm proud of my foray into casual sex. It taught me a lot about myself. And about penises.

That being said, as we talked and he told me about his traditional job and even more traditional life, I thought that even though I was on the square side of hexagonal, after that year, I still might be too alternative for him.

But I kept talking to him. There was something about his affect that calmed me.

His voice was slightly melodic and he gesticulated slowly as he talked, like he had all the time in the world to say whatever he had to say, but maybe he didn't have to say it at all. He listened intently and often took a moment to consider his answers, which was almost jarring in its old-fashioned charm.

---

5   Let's be honest—one of them was a dating rite of passage. The other was because he was attractive and funny and staying in a really nice hotel and my car was locked up in a parking garage. I hadn't discovered Uber yet and I hate cabs. Also, I like fucking.

6   According to a recent survey, the average person in the United States has 7.2 sex partners during his or her lifetime. I imagine the .2 is dry humping?

Who considers anything anymore?

He told me about his daughter, who was studying nursing.

"I'm trying to steer her away from that," he said.

"Why?" I asked.

"Well, she's a really good musician," he said. "She plays guitar and writes her own songs."

"Oh," I said. "So you're trying to convince her to become a musician?"

"Yeah," he said. "She wants to become a nurse, get established, save some money, and then do the music thing. I think that's backward—she should do the music thing now, while she's young and adventurous."

"You realize you're breaking the dad code by telling her that, right?" I asked. "What's she gonna fall back on?"

"I don't know," he said. "My 401(k)?"

Maybe he wasn't quite as traditional as I'd thought.

After we shut the bar down, he said he'd walk me to my car. I told him he didn't have to do that, largely because the week prior, I'd knocked the driver-side mirror off my car coming out of a parking garage and I didn't want him to see it dangling there like the injured appendage of a child whose mother was too irresponsible to take her to the hospital.

He said it was late and it wasn't the best neighborhood, so I grudgingly let him. I stopped short of the front of my broken car to say good night so he couldn't walk me to the driver's door.

He kissed me, sweetly, and it was intoxicating to have to tip my head back so far.

Apparently, I have a thing for tall men. How embarrassingly banal of me.

"I'd like to do this again if you're amenable," he said as he backed away under the glow of a streetlight.

"Oh, I'm amenable," I said as I got into my car and closed the door carefully so the dangling appendage wouldn't whack the door.

He nodded and smiled, then turned and walked away, looking like a figure in an Edward Hopper painting.

That was a good date, I thought as I drove away. *Not earth-shattering. Not "I saw him and I just knew." Just good, warm, and sweet, like I'd been cold and someone put a blanket over my shoulders.*

I thought there might be something there, which I almost never thought. So it sort of was earth-shattering in its non-earth-shattering-ness.

He texted me the next day to ask me out again. I agreed and he suggested a very expensive restaurant in downtown Portland that I definitely couldn't afford on the nonprofit salary I'd been paid for the past decade. But since he'd sneakily paid for the first date while I was in the bathroom, I figured he'd pay for this one, and I thought, *Hells yeah! I'll go to that swanky restaurant with an amazing view and appetizers I can't pronounce! Hooray for archaic patriarchal customs that only made sense when women weren't in the workforce!*[7]

We went and had another lovely evening during which he talked about the friends he'd lost when his first marriage ended, and I talked about the friends I'd lost because I was a jerk.

---

7   Please be on the lookout for my second book, *Of Course I Made Him Pay, I'm No Dummy: Making Sexism Work for You!*

When the check came, I reached for my credit card just to be polite, and tragedy struck: He didn't insist on paying. I'd made a classic miscalculation in assuming he was a "men always pay" guy when in actuality he was a "men always pay unless women offer to pay half, in which case they should totally pay half because, duh, it's only logical" guy.

As the waiter took our cards, I made polite conversation while trying to calculate which bills I wouldn't pay that month. (I would later post about this experience on Facebook, garnering over a hundred and fifty responses ranging from *Never see that cheapskate again!* to *Why did you pull out your card? Rookie move.* I was ambivalent. I love when men pay because I'm usually poor, but I know that if I had money, I'd hate it because it doesn't make any damn sense. My bank account had turned me into a bad feminist.[8])

He drove me home and we made out at my front door, but I didn't ask him in. I wanted to try the "third-date sex = marriage material"[9] theory out on him.

On our third date, we went to a movie. I chose it, and I chose badly. I'd heard *Foxcatcher* was good. I knew it wasn't an uplifting story, but I didn't know exactly what it was about. Pro dating tip: Watching an unrelentingly dark, creepy film based on the true story

---

8   Women who are in favor of men always paying—I get it. I know why you want to fight for this. I love it, too, but it really is illogical. If you truly want equality, you need to let go of this antiquated tradition. If anything, have the waiter split the check so that you pay 40 percent and he pays 60 percent, which makes up for the fact that you make eighty cents for every dollar he makes.

9   To be clear, I didn't want to marry this guy at this point, it's just that my have-sex-immediately tactic hadn't been working, so why not try something new and different? Or, actually, really old and different.

of the 1996 (spoiler alert) *murder* of an Olympic wrestler is not an aphrodisiac.

After the viewing, we both rode the escalator down to the street level at the theater with the glazed looks one might have after watching a man get murdered by Steve Carell, who had seemed so nice on *The Office.*

"Jesus cripes," I said. "I need a drink."

"Excellent idea," he said.

We walked from the theater to a nearby bar, where I apologized for my choice and we attempted to shake it off.

Perhaps because I felt that I had nothing to lose after that movie choice, I told him some of my harder-to-tell stories that night. The story of how I waited way too long to have sex for the first time. How I went to school in New York City and still managed to have a kind of boring time in college because I was afraid of everything. How I'd been heartbroken after my first breakup because my brain hoarded shitty experiences for way longer than other people's did, like those kids who could make their Halloween candy last until summer. I hated those fucking kids.

I was in the middle of telling him all about Build-Your-Own-Burrito Night at the sex club and how upset I'd gotten when they ran out of tortillas when I finally stopped myself.

"What am I doing?" I said. "That's the kind of story you tell someone you never want to see again."

He laughed. "No, that's the good stuff," he said. "Plus, it sounds like you've gotten most of your mistakes out of the way now, so dating you should be a breeze."

"I hadn't thought of that," I said. "I should put the fact that I've met my lifetime mistake quota in my profile. Seems like a selling point."

"Depends on who's reading it," he said. "Some men hope to be your next big mistake."

He seemed unflappable, which was a nice counterpoint to my own perpetual flappability.

We stepped out of the bar and walked to his car in the wet chill of the ever-present Portland mist. He took my hand as we stepped into the street, interlacing his fingers with mine.

The gesture felt quiet and small and monumental.

He drove me home and I invited him in. I offered him a bourbon and we sat on the couch and talked while intermingling body parts before indulging in what can only be described as a colossal make-out session, which led to some extremely hot third-date sex.

He was, miraculously, tender and sweet *and* rough and filthy.

I was smitten.

Not because of the sex (although that helped), but because he was just...good.

I knew he was interesting when we first met. I didn't know how hard and fast I would fall for his curiosity and kindness and how hanging out with him was like having my own personal walking Wikipedia and how easily he took my hand—how it felt warm and simple and real and earnest—and then there was his fucking tallness. He was just. So. Tall.

I know that shouldn't matter, but sometimes a lady has a tall shelf she needs something fetched from. It's very handy.

After our third date, we hadn't really discussed anything serious and I had no idea where this was going, but I knew I didn't want to date anyone else.

We dated for another month, well into February, and my affection for him grew.

It was still too early to have "Where is this going?" conversations, but one night as we sat on my bed, I did note that there was a large gray pachyderm in the room, and I addressed it.

"You just got separated four months ago," I said.

"I did," he said.

"And I spent a whole year dating kind of a lot of people," I said.

"Don't brag," he said. "It's unseemly."

"I'm serious," I said. "You had two single months after ten years of marriage and you can't have sown all the oats you probably wanted to sow."

"I don't think I had that many oats to begin with," he said.

"All I'm saying is, I'm pretty much done," I said. "And you've just begun. Just seems like bad timing."

"I wouldn't say that," he said, scooting closer to me on the bed. "I'd say it's an extraordinary piece of good luck. And I'd be an idiot not to take advantage of it."

That was enough for me. I didn't mention it again.

One afternoon a few weeks later, after putting a two-dollar-and-seventy-five-cent charge on my debit card and incurring a forty-dollar overdraft fee, I was trying to create a budget for myself. I opened Excel, and my dating spreadsheet came up in my Recent Documents. I clicked on it and my stomach dropped.

What the hell had I been thinking? A *spreadsheet*? Really?

It felt especially callous now that there was someone I truly cared about on the list.

He'd scored quite high when I'd first added him, but he hadn't been at the very top.[10] I realized that was because there were some important categories I'd left out, like thoughtfulness, physical affection, being half awake and making a sweet "Mmm" noise whenever I made him the little spoon, and an encyclopedic knowledge of Gerald Ford's 1975 Halloween Massacre cabinet reorganization.

The spreadsheet was such a giant dick move. I was a grown-ass woman, not a frat-boy villain in a John Hughes movie.

But more important—it was ineffectual. Even if I could've accurately predicted my compatibility with someone when I first met him, our feelings about people change as we get to know them. For example, the following week, #28 revealed a new skill that endeared him to me even more: he was an excellent spider killer, and he squealed like a little girl while doing it. Utilitarian *and* entertaining.

Moving forward, I'll only use spreadsheets to create budgets that I'll never stick to, and I'll live with the questionable judgment of my broken head and heart. Because love isn't quantifiable and if we're really smart about it, the last thing we're doing is keeping score.

---

10   That spot was reserved for someone I never saw again after our first date. Anyone can be amazing and perfect when you don't know a goddamned thing about him.

Fellatio Class:

Wherein I Learn That There Are Ways in Which My Oral Fixation Makes Me an Overachiever

It looked more like a museum store than a sex shop. The toys were brightly colored, beautifully sculpted pieces of filthy modern art, and the docent was one pleasant, discreet employee who could talk about the differences among ten different lubes with the same casual friendliness a Whole Foods employee displayed when chatting about olive oils.[1]

They had pushed most of the display tables to the sides of the small shop in order to accommodate the thirty or so students. Among these

---

[1]   Who needs a lube docent? Turns out we all do. Here's what I learned in my five-minute conversation: Use water-based lubes with condoms (*not* oil-based!), but if you're playing in water, use a silicone-based lube, which is the longest lasting, but not if you're using a silicone toy because it'll bond with the surface and make it gummy—in that case, use an oil-based lube, but only if you're not using condoms later. It felt like the most complex if/then statement we'd never learned in high school.

were single women in their thirties and forties who looked like they'd just come from work, two slightly older straight couples, and a few men in their forties who didn't seem to be together. All the students, including me, appeared to be completely engrossed in whatever was happening on their cell phones. Smartphones are a great way to connect with people remotely, but they're also the perfect way to pretend humans aren't actually a thing.

I wriggled to try to find the sweet spot in my metal folding chair[2] and did a little deep breathing to counteract my being-alone-in-a-public-place brain trigger. It doesn't manifest as anxiety so much as a powerful desire to bolt. In this situation, the discomfort was at an 11. So high that my leg seemed to have its own motor.

Our professor was M. Makael Newby, an extremely animated relationship coach and dance instructor who described herself as having a "particular skill for breaking physical action into components and teaching them with enthusiasm." This was not false advertising. Newby is also the author of a choose-your-own-adventure-style erotic novel, which, it turns out, is a literary genre. (Hers has forty-eight unique endings, which is a choice we never get in real-life sex. I have generally experienced one of two endings: having an orgasm or faking one because I feel guilty for taking so long, especially when I'm only exacerbating that issue he has with his neck.)

Before the class began, Newby offered up ten dildos for the bravest among us to practice with, claiming that "muscle memory is a huge part of learning." She had a point, and trying new things was my raison d'be-here, so I raised my hand. She gave me an incredibly realistic

---

2 Metal folding chairs do not have a sweet spot.

flesh-colored silicone penis with the length and girth of a healthy but-
ternut squash and the consistency of a pencil eraser. I thought this
would be helpful if my next boyfriend were the spawn of the Jolly
Green Giant and Gumby.[3]

I held my practice penis in my lap, watching in horror as it grazed
the upper thighs of a latecomer squeezing past me to get to her seat. I
had no idea how to apologize, so I just pretended it never happened,
much like I'd done with all the other humiliating sexual encounters in
my life.

Newby stood at the front of the class next to a wooden bench.
Standing on this bench was her demonstration volunteer, a young,
equally enthusiastic blond woman in her twenties wearing the most
adorable black-and-gold-lamé striped tap pants and a strap-on with a
long, glow-in-the-dark dildo attached.[4] The class communally agreed
to pretend this was just a standard Tuesday night.

So how did I come to be holding this Gumby schlong? you might
ask. A couple of months prior, I'd noticed a class offering in the
newsletter of She Bop, a woman-friendly sex shop in Northeast Portland. The class was called Full-Bodied Fellatio: The Art of Giving
Great Head, which I found right alongside the ad for Bon Appétit!
The Fine Art of Cunnilingus.

At this point, I was a few months into my dating spree (I hadn't yet
met #28), and I was always looking for ways to improve my brand

---

3 I realize it would be impossible for the Jolly Green Giant and Gumby to have
   a child who bears both their DNA because they're both male. Also, they're
   imaginary.
4 Evidently, Newby had used her male partner as a model for some of her classes
   early on, but since the class was an hour and a half long, you can imagine how
   that might be difficult to . . . sustain.

differentiation. I already enjoyed fellatio, but this could be a way to tip me into the eightieth or ninetieth percentile of blow-job-givers. And a class wherein I would sit in the room with a bunch of strangers practicing fellatio fit perfectly into my discomfort zone, so it was also ideal for the OFW Project.

So there I sat, member in hand, waiting impatiently for an opportunity to use it. *I guess this is what it's like to be a man,* I thought.

The class began when Newby passed out the syllabus, which contained headings like Hand Skills, Dry vs. Wet, Playing with Balls!, and, my personal favorite, Introduction to Assholes, which, weirdly, wasn't about my first advertising creative director.

She began with some basics, like the fact that positive reinforcement is far better than negative when it comes to any sort of instruction for sexual partners. This was a real lightbulb moment for me. "Don't do that" gives the other person a million other wrong choices to make. "Do this" gives him one right choice. Take note, mean PE coaches of America.

Then came Hand Skills, wherein we learned that a really good blow job isn't solely a blow job, because you should be using your hands as an extension of your mouth. So think of it more as a bland-job. Or a hojob. There's probably a better portmanteau for it, but you get the idea.

In order to demonstrate this, Newby turned to her tap-panted compadre, put her "penis" into her mouth, and did a series of twists, rotations, and finger gymnastics in addition to the sucking that redefined the term *multitasking.*

I went to take notes and realized that my mouth had dropped open.

I also realized that I wasn't sure what sort of notes I could've written beyond *Do a bunch of stuff.*

It wasn't that she wasn't clear in her instruction. She was. My brain just needed a moment to bridge the gap between *live sex show* and *class*. Don't get me wrong—she was totally professional, as was her demonstration partner. It was by far the least lurid blow job I'd ever seen. But it was still jarring to see a woman enthusiastically sucking another woman's dick and then breaking down each of the choices she'd made into digestible tidbits.

Part of me wanted to look around at my classmates to see if they'd acclimated yet, but the other part of me never wanted to look my classmates in the eyes. Like, ever.

It took a while, but finally, about twenty minutes in, as I was taking notes on ball work, my shoulders dropped down almost to shoulder height and I was able to focus.

The next section on penis basics made me wish I'd paid a lot more attention in health class.

After Newby deep-throated the dildo as she faux-fingered the perineum and I put on my best no-big-whoop face, she dropped some seriously important schlong knowledge on us.

"A lot of people think deep-throating is really important," she said. "But men don't have a lot of feeling at the bottom of the shaft. The majority of the nerve endings in the penis, about eighty percent of them, are in the head and the frenulum—the bit of skin on the underside that connects the shaft to the head."

This didn't make any sense to me. In my (not extensive) experience, deep-throating someone was a sort of blow-job denouement move—a great, dramatic moment that pulls everything together.

Done properly, it generally garners a gasp or two. So how can it be that it's not the most physically pleasurable thing you can do for a man?

But then I thought about the enthusiasm required to do it and re-alized the gasp probably wasn't a response to the sensation so much as to the degree of sexual pluck it took to perform it. This proves that old adage that the most important sexual organ is the brain. (Right after the penis or clitoris.)

I don't want to give away her whole class (you can purchase a PDF of the key points online), but she did give us one more piece of information that I found sort of mind-blowing: If you have the afore-mentioned sexual pluck but your hair-trigger gag reflex has precluded deep-throating, you're in luck. Turns out you can desensitize your gag reflex over time if you're motivated enough. So if you gag at the dentist or when you're brushing your tongue or when you get too close to your boyfriend's balls after he's had a tough workout, you can remedy the first two over time simply by practicing. (The third can be remedied with a shower and a boyfriend sensitive enough to never let you near dirty balls.)

You shouldn't practice on your partner—this would take too long and might start a fight if he claims you're not "applying yourself." The easiest way is to use your toothbrush for ten seconds a night, going farther back each time you get comfortable with a new area. Even-tually, your tongue will be bacteria-free, and your boyfriend will lie there knob-smacked by your new skill.

It truly is a relationship résumé builder.

After this revelation, Newby took us through the rest of the syl-labus with a combination of professionalism and much-needed humor, demonstrating every technique on her assistant, including a finale wherein she ran through about ten techniques in quick succession. I felt like giving her a standing ovation when it was over, but the giant dildo in my lap prevented it.

All the skills were great, but I have to say my favorite moments were less about the mechanics and more about communication.

Newby told a surprisingly heartwarming story about testing her gag reflex with a partner. She'd been going at it for a while, and at one point she went a bit too far, barely avoiding throwing up on his penis but not avoiding throwing up in her mouth a little before running out of the room.

She returned minty fresh, embarrassed, and apologetic, saying, "Sorry. That's *so* not sexy." Her partner smiled sweetly and replied, "Well, I guess we've discovered something one of us doesn't find sexy."

The message being: People make a lot of assumptions around what's "normal" in the bedroom. You think you know what your partner thinks is sexy, which positions you look hottest in, the exact right amount of time it should take to have an orgasm. And when those things don't quite work out (and they inevitably don't), you think your partner is probably disappointed. You're probably wrong. In this case, her partner didn't necessarily find vomit hot (although some people do—more power to you, emetophiliacs!), but he did find it hot that his girlfriend would suck his dick with so much gusto as to almost lose her lunch in his lap.

I once had a friend whose boyfriend liked her to throw pies at his genitals, so that should be more than enough proof that you never, ever know what someone's going to find sexy. (To answer your question, no, I never asked what kind of pies or whether she needed to bake them herself or if something from Safeway would suffice. I'll always regret not asking her, because those are the only two questions people ask when I tell that story. I did once ask her what it was like to date someone with a pie fetish, and she answered, "It's okay, but, y'know...just once I'd like to have sex without putting down a tarp.")

By the end of class, my brain was full and my ass was gloriously happy to get out of that metal chair. I stood up with my classmates and we all filed out, smiling sheepishly as we held our dildos on our way to return them.

"It must be fun washing all these after a class," I said to Newby when I reached her.

"Oh, I just throw them all in the dishwasher," she replied.

I imagined that load—a multicolored garden of dildos sprouting up in rows on the top rack. Mine was definitely a lower-rack item, though.

Even after ninety minutes, I still couldn't totally shake the self-consciousness of being there, like my very presence in the room was an overshare. These are the situations where I have to remind myself that no one is paying attention to me. I know it doesn't sound like a self-care technique, but it is. At certain moments, *No one gives a shit* is one of the nicest things you can say to yourself.

I walked away from the class feeling like I had acquired some good, solid strategies for moving up in the highly competitive world of fellating, and I was eager to try out my skills on some of my partners.

In the months following the class, I didn't see a huge difference in the responses I was getting, but to be perfectly honest, it wasn't as if there had previously been a problem. (I recommend all men date women with a bit of junk in their trunk—odds are, those women have an oral fixation, and that can only work to the men's advantage.) I also hadn't really studied that hard, so there was only a light peppering of Newby's techniques in the mix. That didn't make for a good comparative analysis.

Cut to March: I'd been dating #28 for three months, and I decided it would be fun (and instructive) to apply the scientific method to my fellating. If I paid more attention and stuck to the syllabus, would it make a difference?

So in the spirit of the OFW Project, I mustered up the courage to ask #28 if he would mind being a guinea pig. I told him that I'd try the techniques I'd learned in class on him, and he could tell me whether or not they worked. Additionally, I'd ask him to tell me exactly what he wanted along the way and I'd do whatever he requested.

That sounds horrible, he didn't say.

We decided he'd come over one Sunday afternoon and we'd go full Kinsey on each other. I was pretty comfortable with him sexually by this point, but even so, I flitted around the house before he arrived, sweating profusely and rearranging pillows he would never notice. I dressed in my sexiest red satin nightgown. Well, it was my only nightgown—I'd bought it to wear as a dress to an event earlier in the year, because who the fuck wears nightgowns?

I drank a shot of whiskey before he arrived and studied my class notes a little. My mind went blank. I couldn't remember any of it.

What was that finger-twisting trick she showed us again? This is gonna be a disaster.

I imagined a pornographic version of the *I Love Lucy* episode in which she and Ethel can't stop the conveyor belt so they just shove a bunch of penises in their mouths, willy-nilly.

That didn't help.

When #28 arrived, I offered him a shot as well. He took it.

He seemed fine.

Happy, even.

Jerk.

It was a little strange to just jump right in before the afternoon light had started to fade, but that's what we did.

I grabbed a pillow and threw it on my bedroom floor. I felt my face flush.

"Okay, then," I said, standing arms akimbo and disturbed by how much I sounded like Frances McDormand in *Fargo*.

He grinned, shook his head, and bent down to kiss me.

It was tough to get through the first part, because every move I made, I felt like I was being analyzed, like this was somehow the defense for my sexual dissertation.

Can you tell me why you decided to lick the balls? I imagined him saying.

But after a few minutes of feeling a little like I was doing this for the first time, I was able to jump in wholeheartedly and enjoy it.

What happened next was revelatory for me.

Not because of any skills I learned in class (I frankly forgot to use a lot of them because I was so discombobulated), but because of one simple act: Asking him what he wanted. It wasn't a thing I normally did—ever, really—but this time, in the interest of science, I did it.

There were at least five things he told me to do that I never would've thought of trying. And they *worked*. Of course they did, because he knew his penis. He'd lived with it for over forty years, and they got along super-well.

I found that once I got past the initial self-consciousness, it was a huge relief to be told what to do. I didn't have to question whether he was going to like it, because if he didn't, well, it wasn't my fault.

Hey—you're the one who asked me to pull down on the shaft and hold it taut while lightly sucking the top. Everyone knows that's not one of my signature moves. If you're not excited, that's on you.

Once he had permission to ask for what he wanted, he couldn't seem to stop, and because revealing sexual needs makes a person feel insanely vulnerable, I felt closer to him with every new filthy act he requested. It was the most intimate and dirty sexual encounter we'd had to date.

You'd think that after that experience, I'd be all about telling my partner every one of my sexual needs. It worked so well! I learned so much!

But if the Okay Fine Whatever Project had taught me anything, it was that learning a new skill or engaging in a new activity didn't magically turn me into a person who would use that skill or engage in that activity. I was still me; I just knew more.

So even though I loved being told what to do sexually, I had trouble imagining that my partners felt the same way. I don't have any problem telling someone my fantasies when I'm asked, but I've always avoided giving my partners directions during the act for fear of seeming bossy or killing the mood.

I don't think I'm alone in this. Asking for what we want sexually is really difficult, especially for women, because I think many of us fear that men will feel emasculated if they're not the ones in control.

Sex is also unique in that there isn't another human interaction wherein each of us believes that the other person should inherently know how to please us.

Imagine if your hairdresser asked what you'd like and you responded, "I could tell you that, but if I did, I'm afraid you'd lose your sense of power as a stylist, and it would take all the fun out of the haircut for me. What I'd like for you to do is start cutting my hair and then attempt to deduce the haircut I want by reading subtle verbal and physical cues that might lead you in the right direction. This may be a slight change in my breathing or an infinitesimal head shift toward your hand. And, just to warn you, I might periodically grab your wrist in frustration if you attempt to use hair products or give me a perm, which, if you're the right hairdresser for me, you should have known I hated without my ever having to say a word."

We recognize that would be ridiculous and illogical, but that's exactly what people do with sex. You tell yourself that in an ideal world, your partner will just naturally want to do what you like—that he or she will be satisfied if you're satisfied. If you have to ask for it, you think, *Oh, he's just doing this now because I asked for it, like a sexual honey-do list,*[5] *and so all the romance is gone.*

But that's a dumb thing to think.

Because if my partner is a loving, giving person, the thing that gets him off most is getting me off, whatever that entails. And what I learned from this surprisingly hot blow-job primer with #28 was that he can't know what that is unless I tell him.

---

5   I cannot tell you how much I hate the term *honey-do list.* Sure, we all need a list of tasks, but making it adorable doesn't change how much cleaning the toilet blows.

Perhaps you don't find it romantic to flat-out ask what your partner wants, but for me, working up the courage to ask my boyfriend an embarrassing question and then having him work through the embarrassment of answering it was incredibly intimate. And romantic. And filthy in the best way.

When it was over, I felt proud of myself for pushing through the weirdness to get to the good part. Normally, when I'm first with someone, I do everything I can to avoid weirdness. Weirdness is bad. It's uncomfortable. It's proof that not every moment between us is going to be perfect. But once you've broken through it, you can get to more and better weirdness.

Which we did.

I still had trouble integrating the lesson I learned about the benefits of being a sexual boss, but I found I could be more sexually open via text and during casual conversation over cocktails. In the ensuing couple of weeks, #28 became very good about banking those learnings for later use.

As for the fellatio (or cunnilingus) class, if you want to improve your oral game, I highly recommend taking one, because even if your technique doesn't improve that much, just taking the class is an act of affection for your partner(s).

Can't afford a class, or think sitting in a room with strangers holding a giant dildo doesn't sound appealing?

Just ask your partner what they want.

And then tell them what you want.

I will if you will.

Adventures in Intimacy:

Wherein I Test the Boundaries of Affection and My Bladder

By April, I'd been seeing #28 for three months.

Because of that, many of my other adventures started to quiet down.

No speed-dating or polyamorous married guys with kids' toys on the guest bed to shove away, and, sad to say, significantly fewer naked people dangling from ropes in sex clubs.[1]

But that doesn't mean I wasn't still exploring new territory.

Between December and April, I grabbed my wrench, strapped on my waders, and began plumbing the depths of emotional intimacy.

Since I had handled things poorly in the past, I decided to do

---

1   Zero. That's how many naked people I saw dangling from ropes from December to April. If you're keeping track, that's a 400 percent decrease in dangling naked people from three months earlier.

some research on relationships. What makes them work? How do you keep from losing yourself? How many times can you tell someone to suck it when he suggests watching *Daredevil* on Netflix before you seem inflexible? These were important questions I needed answered.

During my how-to-relationship travels, I stumbled on one of those ubiquitous listicles. You know, the kind that breaks everything down to just a few steps or truths, like "The 10 Things Your Facebook Friends Are Doing That Make Them Actual Adults, Loser" or "3,765 Easy Steps to Finding Love." This one was on a site called Mastering Relationships, which was what I wanted to do.

According to the Relationship Masters, there were seven levels of intimacy in a relationship.

1. Sharing clichés and superficialities
2. Sharing facts
3. Sharing ideas and opinions
4. Sharing hopes and dreams
5. Sharing feelings
6. Sharing weaknesses and fears
7. Sharing needs

The list made me laugh out loud.

As this book clearly illustrates, I am a bit of an oversharer, so I usually leaped from "sharing clichés and superficialities" to "sharing my darkest and most unnerving confessions" during the first date.

Someone could make a lot of money selling shock collars to daters.

You could program in a certain phrase, like *heroin overdose, short prison stay,* or *mashed-potato codependency,* and as soon as the first couple of syllables came out of your mouth, you'd get a shock.

Get on it, science!

So I'm known to leap past levels, but, more impressive, three months into my relationship with #28, I actually created a level all on my own.

I call it the bladder-oversharing level.

One night in early April I was making dinner at #28's house. Lucky for me, he was used to cooking for two kids and didn't have a history of foodies in his past relationships, so my cooking struck him as *interesting* and *exotic* and *not-pizza.* As the smell of red curry and Thai basil wafted through his kitchen for probably the first time ever, I felt like a culinary ambassador.

He was standing in the kitchen with me, leaning on the counter and chatting as I cooked. It was a deeply domestic scene, and the significance of it wasn't lost on me.

At one point, he said something funny. At that same moment, tragically, I happened to be gnawing on a chunk of baby carrot. I proceeded to inhale a relatively large chunk of carrot, which caused me to start coughing. And not just small, ladylike coughing but the kind of full-body hacking that happens when your esophagus believes it's in a life-or-death struggle with a vegetable.

And that's when it happened.

I pretty much peed my pants. (I was wearing a skirt, but you get the idea.)

It wasn't one long pants-peeing but a series of smaller cough-induced urine explosions that soon escaped the bounds of the urine-soaked crotch area until it wasn't just a pants-peeing anymore, it was a shoes-peeing.

One would think that in a situation like this, I'd be with my esophagus—just straight up putting all my energy into surviving this carrot battle—but all my brain could think was *Did I just fucking pee on my boyfriend's floral kitchen mat? Did that just happen?*

He asked me if I was okay and could he help and could he get me some water and I kept shaking my head no as if to say, *Don't come near me! I'm a monster.*

Finally, the coughing fit ended.

I stood there in my pee shoes and wished for a teleportation device that never came.

"Do you need anything?" he asked.

I don't know, I thought. *Adult diapers? A pressure washer? A time machine so I can go back and tell four-years-ago-me to do more Kegels?*

At this point I was still in denial about him finding out; my mind raced with ways that I could distract him long enough to get upstairs and shower.

Should I start a fire? I could start a small one—not big enough to do any real damage, just big enough so that the cleanup would take approximately twenty minutes. I wonder what percentage of house fires are started by people who just peed their pants and are trying to cover it up.

I finally decided I had to tell him because the small pool of urine at my feet was going to give me away no matter what. I mean, unless the entire kitchen was engulfed in flames.

"Um. Underwear?" I responded. "Pretty sure I just peed my pants."

Ah, intimacy.

Those memorable thresholds we cross, like the first kiss, the first time you cry in front of your partner, and the first root-vegetable-induced bladder explosion.

So here it is. Here's the first moment that I can't hide my humanity from you, no matter how hard I try.

I thought back to the reasonably well-dressed and well-spoken bon vivant I'd presented myself as on the second date. That was such a cute skirt. It didn't have any pee on it.

I remembered the social butterfly I became when he met all my friends on Valentine's Day.

And then there was the decent cook who enjoyed a good laugh, the person he'd known just three minutes before.

Dead. They were all dead.

Or not *dead*, exactly, but definitely flailing around on the wet kitchen floor and needing to be woven into a new, incontinent version of me.

He ran upstairs to get me a pair of his boxer-briefs, which I knew wouldn't look as sexy on me as they did on Justin Bieber, so I was going to turn them down.

I went into his guest bathroom and took off my wet underwear while he was gone and (I'm sorry about this, I really, really am) put them in my purse.[2] Thankfully, there wasn't enough collateral damage to my skirt to make it unwearable. I pulled it off, put my foot into the sink, splashed water all the way up my leg and onto the floor in another puddle, then did the same with the other foot. I used his hand

---

2 Yes, I know it's bad, but y'know what? *You* pee all over your boyfriend's kitchen floor, and then I'll allow you to judge me. If it makes you feel any better, I was able to wrap the nonwet parts pretty well around the wet parts. But it was still disgusting.

towel to dry... everything and then refolded it and put it back on the towel rack so that the unused side was available to future guests who hadn't peed themselves.

When I emerged from the bathroom, he offered me the boxer briefs and asked again if there was anything he could do. I told him to stay out of the kitchen for a couple of minutes and he went and sat on the couch. I cleaned up the floor and the floral kitchen mat using paper towels and Lysol, wondering why his kitchen didn't have a bio-medical waste-disposal unit.

All the while, I was wondering how one brings sexy back after an incident like this. Justin Timberlake probably never peed his pants while making dinner for Jessica Biel. I mean, what am I, eighty? Or rather, what is my vagina, eighty? ("I'm not eighty, but my vagina is!"—Worst pickup line ever.)

Three months is a significant moment in a relationship. It's often that fish-or-cut-bait point, where you've gotten semiserious but not totally serious, when you start to think, *I've already invested three months in this. Is there enough there to invest more, or should I come up with an escape plan?*

Complicating matters during this time is that you're still deeply in the limerence phase of love. This is a word coined by psychologist Dorothy Tennov to describe that phase of love where you're still ob-sessed with the other person—his desires, his feelings, what it feels like when he touches you, what he'll look like in a tux on your wed-ding day. It's that one to two-year phase when you're not thinking clearly because your neurons are all clogged with lust and misguided hope. Limerence is probably why some relationships that are doomed last a bit longer than they otherwise would.

But if anything can break through the fog of limerence, it's a splash of pee.

This is what was going through my head as I finished cooking dinner and we chatted.

> HIM: Anyway, I think we'll be able to get the project back on schedule, as long as things go smoothly this week.
>
> MY BRAIN: *I'm sorry... I didn't hear what you just said. I peed my pants earlier.*

I was distracted for most of the remaining food prep—to the point that I'm lucky to still have all my fingers—but then we finished cooking and sat down and had a lovely meal, and I forgot a little. (Give me the right entrée, and I'll forget I accidentally ran over someone with my car.)

Then we retired to the couch, where we chatted some more, made a couple of hilarious adult-diaper jokes, then made out. So he must've forgotten a little too.

It turns out, sexy did come back, and just a couple of hours later.

The only way I can explain it is that I was dating someone who liked humans.

I woke up the next morning and cooked breakfast without incident. I looked across the table at him as I ate my eggs and realized that while I wasn't planning on testing the boundaries of his affection for me like that again, I almost definitely would. Again and again, against my will.

Why do I know this?

Because I once put a tiny candy bar down my pants so I wouldn't eat it.

Because I cry when I get angry, which makes me angrier.

Because I like John Denver. Unironically.

These are bombs that are just waiting to go off someday. And they will go off.

Relationships are all fun and games until someone pees her pants or likes John Denver.

And that's where the real intimacy begins—when you realize the other person can forgive, disinfect his kitchen, and move on with his affection for you largely intact. And when that happens, your affection for him grows because of it.

I think falling in love is half attraction to the best parts of someone and half gratitude for that person's ability to forgive the worst parts of you.

Whatever the reason, we seemed to be falling for each other, so if you're looking for relationship advice, I'm kind of an expert now. I just tell people to buy a family-size can of Lysol and hope for the best.

The MRI:

Wherein I Go on a Medical Adventure of My Own Making and It Is Louder Than Expected

Turning forty has so many perks.

Crepey skin. Back problems. Crushing regret.

But my favorite perk by far is the thing most of us see happening to our parents—you know, the ones who refer to Kiefer Sutherland as "Southern Kieferland."

It's called mild aphasia—or word-finding issues—and it happens to some degree to all people as they age.

I noticed it for the first time while doing a weekly guest spot on a popular Portland podcast called *Cort and Fatboy*. The title sounds like the show had a lot of *ah-ooga!* horns and fart noises, but it was actually quite smart.

It was a pop-culture/sci-fi/"Why did this TV reboot ruin my childhood?" podcast, and Bobby, aka "Fatboy," the producer of the show, was an encyclopedia of arcane pop-culture knowledge. If you were trying to come up with a name, all you had to say was something like "Oh, you know…the kid from that show with the kids and the other kid died of an overdose?"

"Johnny Whitaker from *Family Affair?*"

Yes. Holy shit.

Compared to him, anyone would feel slow on the uptake, but in the beginning I thought I could hold my own.

After a year or so, I noticed that I was stopping a lot to ask for movie titles and I would get caught mid-quip because the name of the person I was lambasting would exit my head forever without leaving a forwarding address.

Oh yeah? Well, tell that to Gary Busey! was what I'd want to quip in response to a crack made by one of the boys.

What would come out was "Tell that to…that guy with the big teeth who got in a motorcycle accident and lost his shit on *Celebrity Apprentice* that one time."

Doesn't have quite the same sting.

At the time, I was still hosting *Live Wire!,* and when you're already anxious about looking like an idiot in front of four hundred people, the fact that you no longer trust your brain makes the situation untenable.

I would research guests for hours, trying to get an angle on them that no one else had, and I'd embed the details of their careers and my questions into my brain so that I'd never draw a blank. But I did draw blanks, despite careful preparation.

What I didn't realize at the time was that, at least in part, the anxiety itself was what was making my brain unreliable.

When you're under stress, your body releases cortisol, also

known as "the stress hormone" and "kind of a dick." I don't mean to disparage cortisol because it does some good jobs, like shutting down unnecessary bodily functions so you can deal with whatever is causing the anxiety. If you have a bear eyeing you like you're his dinner, for instance, cortisol tells your digestive system to stand down for a while so that your more important survival techniques—such as running like the dickens—can have all the resources they need.

However, the downside of cortisol is that it erodes away the synapses—the connections between the neurons—in the prefrontal cortex, which is where the brain houses short-term memory.[1]

Ever notice that you're least likely to remember where you left your keys those times when you're in a massive hurry? And if you're nervous on a date, you suddenly can't remember the name of your second child? (*"I'm pretty sure it starts with an L...or maybe a P? Anyway, it'll come to me eventually. Let's talk about you!"*)

You can thank cortisol for that shit.

Like I said—kind of a dick.

And because of the weekly dread ball that grew in my chest every time I hosted *Live Wire!*, cortisol and I became very well acquainted.

The show always featured comedy—original sketches, stand-up comics, essayists, and interviews, which very often took a humorous

---

1 This was discovered in a University of Iowa study done on older rats, which leads me to wonder, How do you stress out a rat? Tell him that his tech stock is plummeting? Put him in a Barbie Corvette and simulate a car accident? I guess what I'm saying is that I'd be a really good scientist.

turn, even with seemingly serious folks like Susan Orlean and Chuck Palahniuk.[2]

As I mentioned in an earlier chapter, it was the interviews that made me the most anxious. Those unscripted moments were when my synapses needed to fire faster than they did in any other part of the show, but, ironically enough, it was that very anxiety that slowed them down to a crawl.

While written work might be well crafted and satisfying in its own way, an off-the-cuff bon mot that hits hard can make the audience feel honored to be there. And the magic of any great improvised performance is that not only is the performer being wildly clever, she's doing it in a situation where she has to push through the murk of increased cortisol. It's an extraordinary talent, and I was able to access it enough to make me good at my job but not enough to make me great.

I started compensating by going deeper in interviews instead of trying to be funnier. It masked the problem but didn't make it go away.

If you're still young and spry and you've never had word-finding issues, fuck you.

I kid. Let me try that again: If you're still young and spry and you've never had word-finding issues, let me explain how it feels.

Imagine that the words in your brain are in a gigantic labyrinthine library, with each word represented by a book spine that, in your

---

2 Fun fact: When Chuck was on the show, our band performed a satirical version of *Fight Club*, called *Fight Club: The Musical*, which we thought was a hilarious idea. Turns out that at the time, David Fincher was in talks with Trent Reznor to create a *Fight Club* rock opera. If you're reading this, Chuck, you're welcome to use our song. You seemed to love it! (Note: He did not love it.)

youth, you were able to pull down and access immediately. Every day, there are more and more of those books that no one reshelved because your neurons have gotten lazy over time, and you have to wander through the aisles to find them because you weren't really paying attention in school when they covered the Dewey Decimal system. You might see the book on a cart someone's pushing away from you, so you run after it. Sometimes you catch up to it, and sometimes you give up and Google it.

This was happening to me on a fairly regular basis, causing me to "Um" and "What's that thing where you..." a lot more, but I wasn't worried enough to do anything about it. Then, in the spring of my OFW year, it got worse.

I wasn't catching up to the cart anymore. Words were no longer at the tip of my tongue or anywhere near it. They were just gone.

And each time another one went away, I became more paralyzed with fear.

You might know this because you're currently reading my book (thank you!), but I *write for a living*. I also perform live all the time.

I felt like I was losing the things that made me, me.

I'd spent most of my time with comedy people in my personal and professional life, so I'd never been *the* funny one. But I was always *one of* the funny ones. Humor was a huge part of how I related to people, and it was disappearing in my daily interactions. Which, not surprisingly, looked a lot like happiness disappearing.

And while this was happening, I felt like my tenure at *Live Wire!* was coming to an end. There had been rumblings of making a smaller, more intimate show and I had a feeling that it probably wouldn't include me.

And as much as that made sense, the idea of making such a seismic shift after twelve years left me feeling completely lost.

So the stress over the show was ramping up at the same time the stress over my memory was ramping up, and the inside of my brain started to feel like an old clock, sometimes running too fast and other times grinding to a halt, usually at the most inopportune moments.

Occasionally, I would lose a word in the morning, the same way any normal, not-nuts woman in her forties does.

But I have generalized anxiety disorder. So as soon as that happened, my anxiety would spike. I started to Google *memory loss* and *word-finding issues*.

Here's a piece of advice: If you're having memory-loss issues, *don't* Google *memory loss*. Go to your doctor. Because absolutely nothing good comes up when you Google *memory loss*. You're not going to hit a page that says, *Sometimes memory loss is caused by an impending lottery win* or *Memory loss could signal the onset of the greatest batch of chili you've ever made in your life.*

Google has wreaked so much havoc on the medical world that there's now an unofficial diagnosis for people who believe they have one or multiple diseases after Googling their symptoms: cyberchondria.

I have this. I spend an inordinate amount of time on WebMD, which I call Pinterest for Hypochondriacs. They just need to let you create boards with your favorite disease families in them, like Dermatological Disorders I Probably Have, New Viruses That Are Definitely Going Around My Office, and Cute Cats That Might Have Given Me the First Human Case of Feline Leukemia.

What diagnoses did my WebMD memory-loss searches lead me to? Early-onset Alzheimer's, dementia, and a brain tumor.

So—the opposite of really good chili.

Each time I'd stop in the middle of a sentence, my chest would tighten, and warm tingles of fear would wash over my whole body.

I'm losing my mind.

I won't be able to write anymore.

How will I make money?

Scott and Mom will have to take care of me.

I won't remember who they are.

I'll become even more of a bitch.

I won't be able to remember all the things I used to hate.

What if I start watching Real Housewives of Atlanta *and enjoying it?*

I finally got my doctor to send me to a neurologist. He gave me a couple of quick tests in his office and didn't seem that worried.

"The good news is you don't have any of the immediate hallmarks of a degenerative brain disease, but if your word loss feels higher than that of your peers, it may be cause for some concern."

The first part of the sentence was completely erased by the second part.

That's how generalized anxiety disorder works. It's like your life is the Godfather series, and all you can see are Sofia Coppola's parts in the third one.

"I think this is probably being caused by your anxiety," he added. "But let's schedule a neurological test anyway, just to be sure."

He was referring to a four-hour neuropsychological evaluation involving remembering stories, numbers, words, and shapes; it's apparently quite accurate in determining whether there's something degenerative at play. Since it's such a long test, it often takes a couple of months to schedule one.

He recommended the test in March, and by June, I still hadn't heard a word from the scheduling team, even after calling repeatedly.

But I handled the wait with great aplomb.

Or—the opposite of that.

Each morning I would get up, and the first word that escaped my already-fretful mind would set off my nerves, but instead of just the usual quiet, nagging unease, I'd walk through the day with a crippling emotional buzzing that distanced me from every detail of my life. It was like living behind bulletproof glass but if the guy with the gun was in there with me. And of course, with more pervasive worry came more word-finding issues, which would then increase the anxiety tenfold until I was just a walking ball of electrified wires.

But I still needed to go to work, and I still needed to try to hang out with my friends and my semi-new boyfriend of five months like a normal person.

Much of my life felt like those moments after smoking weed with my workmates. It was like I was in a movie scene where people were talking but I couldn't hear them; I could only see their mouths moving in slow motion while my brain whirred out of control.

"You look cute today."

Thanks. I'm probably dying.

"Do you have the show rundown finished?"

I would, except that my brain isn't working anymore and I'll never have a job again and then I'll die.

"Do you want to go out or cook tonight?"

Let's cook because I won't be able to do it for much longer and then we'll have to break up because we just started dating and you're not going to want to start feeding me and reminding me of what medications to take and doing that thing Ryan Gosling did in The Notebook *where you write the whole history of our relationship of five months in a, well, notebook, because there wouldn't be that much in it except for a lot of sex and us going to comedy shows and me peeing on your floor.*

One Saturday in May, after a particularly difficult memory week, some things went sideways at a *Live Wire!* show. I'd screwed up the seating for some important guests, a cooking segment I'd produced had proven far more complicated than I'd imagined, and I wasn't feeling confident about an essay I was about to perform. This was all pretty standard stuff that normally I'd just deal with, move on, and chalk up to another night in the glamorous world of public radio. But during that period, I was starting each day frazzled, so by the time the show began that evening, I was already on the bumpy road to full-on decompensation.

Adding to my agita was the fact that #28 had come to see the show, as he had every show since we started dating, and I wasn't thrilled at the prospect of reading my essay and embarrassing myself in front of him. Some may ask, "After what happened in his kitchen, how could anything you did onstage possibly be worse?" You'd be surprised at how much more humiliating bombing onstage can feel compared to a nice, intimate pants-peeing. Just take your last mortifying incident—say, getting caught by another driver picking your nose. Now imagine that was a clown car filled with hundreds of people. It feels a little worse, right?

I sat at the producers' table, and as the show progressed, the urge to cry kept popping up at inopportune moments, like during a stand-up comic's set or when Luke was doing his monologue or right before I read my essay. The show had just moved to Revolution Hall, a much larger venue than we'd been in the previous season, and the producers' table sat in front of seven hundred and fifty audience members, as did the stage I stood on to perform my essay. So during the show, I was protected by the natural human disinclination toward self-mortification. My essay went fine, as it always did—a fact my brain never seemed to learn even after over a decade of performing them.

To my great relief, the tears didn't come. That is, until the show ended. They came at the exact moment the band started playing the theme music. It was as if that was the floodgate-opening cue. There was nowhere for me to go. The theater was filled with fans, cast, crew, and, even worse, guests whom I couldn't let see me like this.

I managed to get out of the building through a side door. I ran to my car and got in, sobbing.

I wasn't crying because of a few fuckups during the show, I was crying because every single day for months I had been imagining losing myself—imagining that I would soon forget every detail of my life and every person in it that ever meant anything to me—and I'd finally cracked. I sat there, drenched in tears and regret and sorrow I hadn't allowed myself to feel all this time because I couldn't have functioned inside it all.

I started the car and left #28 at the theater.

I got a few blocks away and got a text from him.

Did you just pull an Elvis? Did you leave the building?

I texted him back.

I'm so sorry. I'm sobbing and it's not pretty and I don't want you to see me ugly-cry.

Let me be clear: If #28 had just up and left me at an event we were both attending, it would've been a break-uppable offense in my mind—at least, immediately after it happened. It was just so overly dramatic.

He was more understanding.

Okay. Well, text me when you get home and we'll talk about it. Drive safely.

I'd finally reached a point where the thing I'd been hiding from him for three months had gotten so bad that it was now most definitely un-hideable.

My boyfriend had a history of relationships with…complicated women, and I didn't want to be another one, which was why I'd downplayed my fears since March.

I'd let him know what they were but didn't tell him that my anxiety was overwhelming and pervasive. That it colored almost every day and every experience. That my fear that I had some degenerative brain disease was the reason I hadn't told him that I loved him.

Five months in, that felt to me like a deal breaker.

When I got home from the show, #28 and I talked on the phone, and even though I didn't deserve it because I was a giant boyfriend-leaving asshole, he calmed me down. He knew a lot about anxiety and depression meds due to his experience with his family and exes.

He was being kind and caring and understanding, but I thought maybe he was just waiting until I wasn't in crisis to dump me. I was sure he had to be thinking, *How the hell did this happen again? Is* nut job *my type?*

The next day, I put my relationship problems on the back burner and e-mailed my neurologist to let him know my symptoms seemed to be worsening. He said that due to the length of the test and staffing issues, the test scheduling was just going to take however long it took, but if I wanted to rule out certain pressing issues, I could get an MRI.

Ruling out pressing issues sounded like a hoot.

So I scheduled an MRI for the following week at 6:30 in the morning.

The day of the appointment, in the most *Valley of the Dolls* moment of my life, I woke up at 5:45 a.m. and immediately took a Xanax.

Xanax is a benzodiazepine and is dangerously addictive, but when you're having a mild anxiety attack, it's like perspective in a pill. Once you've taken it, all those thoughts that used to be racing are now sitting quietly drinking tea and reading the latest Nordstrom catalog.

This wasn't a mild anxiety attack, though. I was still the aforementioned ball of electrified wires, but the Xanax helped to keep the voltage below about two hundred.

My brother came to pick me up at 6:15 and we drove out to the hospital in Clackamas, a suburb of Portland that's just as uncharming as its hard-consonant-filled name suggests.

I put on a gown and went into the room with the machine.

The MRI is a highly advanced machine that creates a strong magnetic field (about a thousand times as strong as a fridge magnet) and uses radio waves to give doctors a 3-D image of what's happening all up in your business.

It looks like a giant doughnut with a tongue.

I lay down on the tongue and the two technicians, Ashley and Rick, talked me through what was going to happen. The tongue would pull the top half of my body inside the doughnut (my words, not theirs) and the machine would make mechanical noises for about twenty-five minutes.

Rick asked me if I was claustrophobic.

Of course I'm claustrophobic, Rick. What kind of generalized anxiety sufferer would I be if I wasn't? I'm not an underachiever, you dick.

I just said yes.

I'd seen people on TV get MRIs and it always seemed strange to me to be claustrophobic when half of your body was out in the open and you could see the rest of the room from where you were lying. It was like freaking out because you were afraid of heights on the first floor.

Rick put my face into a plastic mask attached to the machine to keep my head from moving. That triggered a mini-freak-out, but it didn't last. It did make me think that Hannibal Lecter would've skated through an MRI. Just another thing to add to his large list of accomplishments.

"Okay, Ashley's going to press a button now, and that will pull you into the machine," Rick said. "Just let us know if you have any issues."

The tongue started moving and I was eased into the doughnut hole, an experience that would've been welcome in a Wonka-like dream (especially if it was a chocolate glazed) but was now presenting a problem.

Nope. No. No-no-no-no-no-no-no-no-no. *Oh no.*

"I need to get out," I said as coolly as possible.

"Okay, she's reversing it, just stay calm," Rick said.

What. The. Actual. Fuck, brain?

How was that scary? There were two feet between my head and

the wide-open space of the hospital MRI room, but that didn't preclude my thinking, *Push that fucking reverse button, Ashley, because I will claw my way out of this miracle of modern medicine if I have to.*

I didn't have to—Ashley got me out and asked impatiently if I had access to more Xanax. I could tell Ashley had met more than her share of MRI scaredy-cats and wasn't having any of this.

My brother handed me another Xanax and I chewed it so it would work faster. Rick and I waited for the new Xanax to kick in while Ashley mentally gave me the finger.

After about twenty minutes, we tried again. Rick said he would stay by my side and he was rubbing the top of my knee, which sounds creepy, but I think they do it so you'll have a physical reminder of the outside world while in the machine.

I got pulled back in and seemed almost okay with it this time.

And that's when the noises started.

As the huge magnets whirred around the machine, they made a high-pitched, repetitive buzzing, like someone was using the world's largest hair trimmer on a giant. That went on for about five minutes before it stopped, and the loud, droning alarm started.

Are we at DEFCON 1? Because if I remember my WarGames *correctly, this is definitely the sound of DEFCON 1.*

Nope. Apparently, that's just another MRI sound.

That ended, and the next sound you're supposed to be cool with was cued up, sort of a *thump, drag, thump, drag,* like a zombie in leg irons approaching.

Am I being punk'd? Rick? Did my brother put you up to this? Because this is hilarious...ly cruel.

Then more repetitive buzzing, then *whack-whack-whack-clang, whack-whack-whack-clang, bump, buzz, whack, clang-whack,* Are you fucking kidding me *whack-clang* with this *clang-whack* shit?

At this point my fear was overtaken by comic glee. (This may have coincided with more of the Xanax kicking in.)

I pictured Ashley in her booth with a bunch of Foley artists with jackhammers, chains, leaf blowers, and DEFCON 1 buzzers, and she was conducting them like an Orchestra of Unsettling Sounds.

So modern medicine has come up with a way for doctors to see into our bodies, but in order for them to do it, patients have to experience what it's like to be inside a running airplane engine.

Twenty-five minutes and 456 fucked-up noises later, I emerged from the machine into the real world.

I gave Rick and Ashley a closed-mouth smile that said, *I'm really sorry. I know it's illogical, but so are a lot of things. Have you ever seen a narwhal?*

So that was the end of the waiting-to-get-the-MRI anxiety.

Now there was just the anxiety of waiting for the results.

About a week later, I got them.

I was shopping with my mother at Bath and Body Works when the e-mail came. I told her the results over a mahogany teakwood candle, which made the moment all the more special.

Clean. No abnormalities, no brain tumor.

As my mother drove me home from our relief-induced candle binge, I did a cursory search on what an MRI can reveal about degenerative brain diseases. Evidence of Alzheimer's generally doesn't show up on a scan until the disease is pretty far advanced. So after all that, the only thing the MRI had ruled out was a brain tumor, and

I was happy about that for fifteen minutes before starting to worry again about what my failing brain might mean.

Once again, welcome to GAD, where happiness is fleeting and holy shit, does this mole look like it's grown to you?

This battle with my brain continued until mid-July, when I finally had my four-hour neurological test.

The test was nerve-racking, what with the future of my brain hinging on the results. It was a long series of puzzles and stories and numbers I needed to repeat back, and as I was taking it, I was sure I was failing miserably. But even though I went through the entire test in the throes of my ongoing anxiety, according to the results, I was fine.

I did have mild aphasia, but apparently, it wasn't due to a degenerative brain disease. It was probably due to GAD.

My obsession about dementia was most likely because the stress of my impending job shift had triggered my OCD, almost exactly on schedule. Just like the previous two episodes, this one happened around a huge change I needed to make in my life but was avoiding. It's a strange thing when your unconscious mind knows you need to do something before your conscious mind does. Also strange to have your brain essentially attack you to force you to make that change.

This episode created intrusive thoughts saying that my brain was dying on me, and the horrible thing about this fear was that I couldn't counteract it with logic.

In past OCD episodes, my fear was always that I'd already hurt someone or that I *would* hurt someone, like I'd randomly grab a knife or a gun and suddenly do something I'd never had the impulse to do before, something that went against everything that I was and that

I believed in. I could reason those fears away with simple questions: Have I ever attacked someone with a knife before? Do I want to do something like that now? Am I a psychopath? (That last one is a little hard to decide for oneself, but since I believe I'm an empathetic person and I didn't watch *American Psycho* and think, *Well, he seems like a nice young man. I wonder if he's single,* I felt like it was safe to assume that the answer to that one was a no.)

But this dementia fear was much more problematic. The symptoms listed online for the diseases I was concerned I had actually supported my neuroses instead of counteracting them. This is why I'm sure doctors wish the internet had never been invented. It's like throwing gas on a smoldering log. A really, really irrational smoldering log. And while it wasn't likely that I was suffering from one of these diseases, it also wasn't completely out of the question in the same way that, say, me grabbing a knife and stabbing my roommate was.

Thankfully, once I got my test results, my brain decided to stand down. After one last gasp of a two-day freak-out when I went off the Xanax, I stopped worrying that I had a degenerative brain disease.

But I learned something from a psychiatrist about generalized anxiety disorder during my three-month stay in Stress Central. I learned that when you have it, even if you're not feeling anxious, your anxiety is free-floating, just hanging around waiting for something to attach to.

I knew that from now on, I needed to manage my anxiety or it would blossom into OCD episodes whenever I went through a big life change like moving, getting a new job, or a death in the family. Not exactly ideal times to have massive, crippling anxiety.

I also knew that what I had to offer #28 might not have been a girl-friend with a degenerative brain disease, but it was a girlfriend with a mental illness that she'd have to manage for the rest of her life.

We were watching the first season of *Fargo* on his couch when I told him that my tests had come back okay.

"Well, that's great!" he said, taking my hand.

"It is great," I said. "I'm relieved, for sure. But my doctor does think that my constant ruminating was probably due to another OCD episode. And it probably won't be my last one."

"Well, there are ways to treat OCD, right?" he asked.

"Sure," I replied. "Medication, cognitive behavioral therapy. Exercise. The usual."

He shrugged. "That seems doable," he said, looking into my eyes and not running or screaming or running and screaming.

I looked at him closely.

"It does," I said. "It does seem doable."

He bent his head down and kissed my hand. "I'm so glad you're okay," he said. "I knew you were really worried. I hated that."

He didn't seem fazed. Of course, he may have been fazed but pre-tending not to be. (I don't want to disillusion anyone, but people in relationships sometimes lie.)

Whether he was fazed or not, his response wasn't to pull away from me.

He pulled me closer. He let me know he was just as relieved as I was that my brain wasn't going to die any time soon and he didn't seem to mind that it was a little broken.

I felt a surge of love for him caused by what was, on the surface, nothing.

I loved him because nothing changed. He looked at me with the same eyes and held me exactly as tightly as before. He had learned my Worst Thing and his response was basically *I'm so sorry you have that Worst Thing and that it brings you pain. Now, what should we have for dinner?*

We were fine.

So we were wonderful.

One Last Leap:

Wherein I Do the Thing I Should've Done Years Ago and Try Not to Wallow in Regret

In the fall, my year of mini-adventures was over, and it was time to start another season of *Live Wire!*[1]

I was beginning my third year as head writer and co-producer of the show while Luke Burbank hosted.

During my tenure in this role, a lot of people asked me what it was like to watch someone do the job that had been mine for a decade.

The answer was: It was unusual, but not unpleasant.

The first time I sat at the producers' table, it felt surreal being on the other side of the speakers, watching Luke talk to the audience that had, just a couple of weeks earlier, been there to watch me. It

---

1   We took summers off because it was virtually impossible to get Portlanders to sit inside during the sun-drenched summers. Then in the fall, we'd start up our comedy show again, just in time to coincide with the arrival of everyone's seasonal affective disorder. Genius!

was like watching a new stepparent with your own kids, if you had hundreds of kids who were all approximately the same age as you and who wore Columbia Sportswear jackets and drank cheap pinot grigio.

Stepping down had been a struggle, and I had immediately wondered how long it would take me to miss hosting.

But I can honestly say that in two-plus years of producing and writing, I never once wished for my old job back. (If you'll recall, I did sit on a toilet in a bar crying missing the things my job had brought me—but I never wanted the job back. I knew what it would have done to me.)

If I had longed to get my job back at any point, all I would've had to do to get rid of that feeling was think of the moments that were crazy-making.

Like the time I thought musician M. Ward was just bashful when he clammed up while I was interviewing him in front of a sold-out crowd, but then he turned his back to the audience and gave me a devilish grin that made me think, *Is he fucking with me right now? I feel like right now is a super-bad time to fuck with me.*

Or the time comedian Mike Birbiglia called out an audience member for sitting in the front row knitting during our interview, also known as a Peak Portland Moment.[2]

---

2   I want to make it very clear that I'm not faulting Birbiglia on this, I'm faulting the audience member who could've chosen anywhere to knit—the back row, the bar in the theater, her living room—but chose the front row of a theater where a live show was being recorded. Afterward, we had one of our fans knit a merkin and send it to Birbiglia with a note saying that this was what the woman in the audience had been knitting. I don't think it fit him because we never got a thank-you note.

Or the time we booked a vintner around the holidays to talk about champagne, and for whatever reason, he walked onstage and did not want to discuss anything about champagne. Maybe he was sick of it. Maybe champagne slept with his wife. I don't know what happened, but it was by far the most excruciating ten minutes of my hosting career.

Listening to the segment again years later, I could actually hear the tension in the audience grow as the interview progressed and he expounded on all subjects decidedly *not* champagne-y with every question I asked. The entire segment turned into an inside joke between the audience and myself during which we all imagined the champagne evasion couldn't possibly last another question...and then it did. Once we got past about the seven-minute mark, the audience roared with laughter at every non-champagne-related answer, which was all of them. I finally ended the interview after I was able to get him to answer one question. He then sabered a bottle of champagne before he left (*sabering* is where expert champagne-bottle openers skillfully pop off the champagne cork, along with the glass bottle lip, simply by running a knife up the bottle with the right amount of force). When he did, the bottle fragment and cork flew into the second row, narrowly missing one of our season-ticket holders.

I'm sure I made some quip at the time, but what was going through my mind was *Why didn't he saber the bottle toward my head so I could be in an ambulance right now?*

But I was no longer host, so those moments of terror/wishing for bodily harm almost never happened.

Except this one time.

It was when sex-advice columnist and pundit Dan Savage was about to go onstage for his interview and we realized that he hadn't approved the sketch we'd sent him to appear in because our producer had forgotten to actually attach the attachment to the e-mail in which she described the attachment, a move I could've sued her for using because that was totally my move.

We'd written Dan some lines wherein he asked our cast for sex advice and they steered him horribly wrong, but Dan didn't consider himself an actor so he was uncomfortable performing lines that he hadn't had a chance to read over.

When I realized what had happened, a soccer-ball-size dread ball immediately arrived. I wasn't prepared for this—one of the reasons one goes into comedy writing is that it tends not to put you in emergency situations.

These were the kinds of moments where struggling with anxiety made me feel like a not-so-great producer. Because more than just about anything, a live producer's job is to appear calm and have a plan no matter what.

There's an improv tenet known as "fit and well" that's really about performing, but it works for anyone who's trying to lead a staff. It is what it sounds like—you come into the situation happy to be there with an open mind and heart, and no matter what happens on or off the stage, you project an unmistakable affect that everything is great and going as planned. If a can light drops from the rig and strikes the announcer on the head, you smile, laugh, and let the audience know it's a gag while you secretly dial 911.

The problem with me appearing fit and well is that my face wears every emotion I have like a sequined gown under disco lights.

In these cases, I think my staff had become used to the fact that even though I might not have been projecting the idea that everything was going to be okay, I would probably find a way to make everything okay regardless. It wasn't an ideal dynamic, but just like we learn to deal with parents who have deficiencies, we learn to work with our flawed managers.

Thankfully, because Mr. Savage was a gracious person, he was willing to read real questions he had about sex and have our cast answer those. In the final minutes before being whisked away to do his interview, Dan wrote five questions on the back of a script page. That meant we had approximately nine minutes to write the cast's responses and get them back onstage.

This seemed like the perfect time for a dread ball to blossom into a full-blown panic attack, but it didn't. What's frustrating about these disorders is how capricious they can be. Sometimes they don't show up when, given the circumstances, they absolutely should (like when you have nine minutes to write what usually takes hours), and sometimes they show up when you wouldn't expect them to in a million years. (Why did my first onstage anxiety attack happen while I was hosting a breakfast for a nonprofit? Talk about low stakes.)

Anyone who works in a high-stress environment will tell you that sometimes fear serves you. If properly harnessed, it allows you to do things you never thought you could. I just generally didn't have a very effective harness. But that night, I did.

I wrangled all our actors together and grabbed two guest writers who were standing at the side of the stage watching the sold-out show and pulled them backstage.

Comedian Jen Kirkman happened to be a guest on that show and she was sitting waiting to go on when the entire creative staff descended on the greenroom.

I read each of Dan's questions one by one, then asked which writer had an idea for how to answer it. The three writers each took one, I took one, and Jen took the fifth one.

Miraculously, because my fear of the show sucking overwhelmed my fear of asking one of my comedy heroes for a favor, I asked Jen if she wanted to write one. She was a huge Dan Savage fan and agreed.

After taking five minutes to write my own response, I went to the writers and asked what they'd come up with. You'd be amazed at how laser-focused a writer can become when faced with impending public humiliation.

Maybe it was great stuff, or maybe we were desperate, but we massaged each answer as much as we could in literally half a minute, and then I gave all the actors their hand-scrawled scripts just before our stage manager called for them.

At the last second, I realized that Dan didn't have his script because we'd been using his to write from, so I ran out onto the stage, slowed down as soon as the audience could see me, and casually handed Dan his script just as Luke was announcing the bit.

More than any other time in my tenure on *Live Wire!*, those nine minutes made me feel like I was in show business. Or, more accurately, like I was in a madcap 1940s picture about show business, where I was the young upstart writer with real moxie who came through in the nick of time.

"See, fellas? Told you we'd get it to ya! Just like my mother used to say—you can always count on a Hameister girl!" [Cue music and credits.]

It wasn't the best bit we ever wrote, but it was by far the most exciting to write. And when Dan asked if cunnilingus was something straight people and lesbians made up just to freak out their gay male friends and Andrew Harris said yes it was (along with Arbor Day, falcons, and pleated khakis), I felt a real sense of pride that we were educating people.[3]

So there were still moments happening—moments that I couldn't have possibly experienced working at any other job, at least not one in Portland—but they were fewer and farther between for me as the show shifted voices and I felt like I had less to say. (You'd be amazed how much verbal ground you can cover in twelve years.)

Which I suppose was a blessing in disguise because after all my mini-adventures were over, it looked like I might be going on another.

During the all-day summer retreat we took every year, the show's executive team (which included me) continued the discussion about the need to scale down in order to get more intimate, in-depth interviews. We'd been in a beautiful seven-hundred-and-fifty-seat venue called Revolution Hall, which was great when we had huge guests, but it made it harder to get those guests to reveal things. When in front of an audience that large in an imposing venue, people tend to want to perform more than they want to engage in a real conversation. And when you have only a limited time with them, this

---

3   We weren't.

can become problematic for getting what they call in radio "good tape."[4]

So, led largely by Luke's vision, the team decided to take the show "down to the studs," a metaphor I assume Luke used because he was doing significant renovations on his house at the time.

No cast, very little pre-written content, since Luke was more of an off-the-cuff guy. Mostly, the show would be Luke interviewing guests with music and periodic comedic interjections from the announcer or a local comic. It would be very much like a staged version of his podcast *TBTL*. It made perfect sense and we should've done it from the very beginning when I first stepped down as host.

But I knew what it meant.

The show would no longer need a head writer.

As I sat there, recognizing that my job was being phased out in what was a surprisingly casual conversation, I knew I shouldn't fight it. The fact was, I didn't have much to offer *Live Wire!* anymore, and it didn't have much to offer me.

When we were about to break for lunch, our moderator, a great friend of the show who was one of the kindest and most intuitive people I knew, weirdly decided to go around the room and ask us what we thought was the most constructive thing we'd accomplished that morning.

"Courtenay?" he asked when he got to me. "What's yours?"

I looked at him, almost speechless as tears welled up in my eyes.

---

4   If you're under the age of thirty, *tape* was a flat piece of plastic coated with ferric oxide that you could record sound onto. This was back in olden times when people used telephones for talking and called each other assholes in person instead of in the comments section of BuzzFeed.

"Can I pass?" I said. "I think I'd like to pass."

Maybe people were being so casual because they knew I wasn't very happy in my job, but I'd worked on the show for twelve years. I'd never done anything for twelve years except age and eat a lot of carbs.

Plus, you know that thing where even if you don't really like your dog, you're still going to cry if it dies after twelve years? I'm not a monster.

The show brought so many extraordinary things and people into my life. It made me a writer. And now it was going away.

If I was honest with myself, I knew it was for the best.

Because after twelve years, I was bored. And a little annoyed.

I shouldn't have been. This little thing we'd started in a tiny theater in an old Portland movie house twelve years earlier was now syndicated by PRI on public radio stations around the country. We'd done the thing we'd always wanted to do, so I should have been happy.

I was annoyed because I was out of ideas. Well, not any ideas as much as big ideas. Show-changing ideas. I was trapped in all the things we'd done in the past and unable to imagine a different show.

I remember thinking, *You can do anything you want. So what do you want to do?*

And the only ideas that bubbled to the surface were things I couldn't do on the show. Screenplay ideas. Podcast ideas. Brownie-recipe ideas. I was in trouble.

Even so, I could've found a way to stay if I had truly wanted to. The show still needed writers, and the other producers suggested I could stay on as a freelancer. I considered it, and a year earlier, I might've taken them up on it. But I was, ever so slightly, different now. The OFW Project had changed me.

Now, complacency and fear didn't have to win.

Now, I said, "The show needs to move on and so do I."

And I don't know that I would've said that if I hadn't had all my mini-adventures: if some small part of my lizard brain hadn't learned over the past year that there was a chance everything was going to be okay.

I had a friend who quit a job he'd been unhappy in after seven years, and a couple of weeks later, he left his decade-long marriage. Neither had been working for him, but he had to take that first leap to know that he'd survive the second one.

I think my story is similar. It's just that instead of taking two big leaps, I took a series of little ones and then one giant one.

I'd written my last column and quietly put the OFW Project to bed just a couple months earlier, but there were clearly some remnants of the "What the hell, why not?" attitude I was sometimes able to muster.

I was proud that I'd done a thing for twelve years that turned into something truly special. But I was even prouder that I'd done a thing for twelve years despite the fact that it scared the shit out of me.

And now I was scared again.

It's scary to leave a shiny beautiful thing for a new thing whose luster level is unclear.

But standing at the end of a diving board wondering if you still remember how to swim isn't a sustainable plan either. Eventually you're going to get cold and need a sandwich.

I worked ten more shows, and I was gone that winter with no earthly idea where I would end up.

So this is one last message for the timid: I'm one of you, and I stepped off.

I didn't dive in, because that's how people crack their heads open. And I can't tell you the water's fine because I have no idea what sort of chemical maintenance this pool undergoes. Plus, it's a public pool, so we're all rolling the dice in that way, but still.

I'd leaped off hundreds of tiny diving boards into tepid little kiddie pools, and that was enough to prepare me for one final, messy cannonball.

I'm a tsunami, motherfuckers.

Deal with it.

The Epilogue That's Really Just
Another Chapter:

Wherein I Attempt to Tell
You Why You Just Read This
Whole Fucking Book

Wondering what happened to me after I left the show? Whether I survived? Whether I started a podcast, like 130 percent of American comedy writers?

I'll tell you, and I did, and I didn't. Yet.

As for my romantic life, I'm still with #28.[1] It's been two years and I still love him and he still loves me and neither of us has slept with a field hockey team so I put that in the Win column.

We've had suspiciously few issues in our relationship, but that's probably because we mostly see each other on weekends and problems don't usually crop up when all you're doing is having sex, going

---

1   His name is Scott. Which is my brother's name. I know it's weird, but if we can deal with it, so can you.

on road trips, and estate-sale hopping. ("Wanna go see dead people's stuff this weekend?" "Always.")

He is an introvert and I wouldn't describe him as effusive, but even so, I haven't had to spend a lot of time wondering how he feels about me. After two years, there's nothing like still hearing "I can't wait to see you" and "I'm so glad you came over tonight." He is devoid of pretense, and for a person whose internal radio is always set to the rumination station, that's quite a gift.

I've continued to struggle with my weight. It's one thing to have body issues when you're single, but being with someone, even someone who has never once mentioned your body size except to make "hubba-hubba" noises about it, exacerbates the problem.

About a year into our relationship, my weight started creeping up again. I found myself ten pounds heavier than I'd been when I'd met him and felt a lot less sexy. For three years I'd been using this app called Lose It to track my food intake, exercise, and weight. The app included an interactive chart that showed your weight over time, so you could scroll back and forth on your timeline and see your weight magically appear on every date you weighed yourself for as long as you'd had the app. I'd had it since 2013, so with just a finger flick, I could witness years of weight obsession, successes, frustrations, diet failures, and rationalizations fly by, date by date.

Some people might look back nostalgically on times in their lives when they were more functional, more hopeful, or just happier. I look back on past weights. I remember when I was twenty and got down to a hundred and thirty-five pounds and a size 10 after paying for a service wherein a "nurse" supervised my three-hundred-calorie-a-day diet for four months. I remember when I was twenty-eight and went from two hundred and twenty-five pounds to one hundred and ninety by walking on a treadmill in my mom's laundry room after my father died. I remember when I was thirty-three and lost seventy pounds because I had finally gained enough self-esteem to believe I deserved to be with someone but not quite enough to believe I could do so while fat.

I have snapshots in my mind from each of these times: Trying on size 10 skirts in the Esprit store and not recognizing myself. Standing in front of a huge crowd in a gorgeous old movie house for *Live Wire!* and feeling sexy and confident for the first time in my life at thirty-four. Then standing on that same stage at forty-six and thinking it was miraculous that all I felt was nervous about my performance instead of worried that people were leaning over to their dates and saying, "She sounds a lot thinner on the radio."

I'd had those affirming, confident moments in the past, so why wasn't I having them now? Here I was, almost as thin as I hoped I sounded on the radio, and in a relationship with a guy who loved me and my body. Why couldn't I love it too?

I'm five foot five, and when we first started dating, I weighed just under two hundred pounds, so I wasn't harboring any illusions that I was rail-thin, but I felt that I had a lot to offer. I was curious and empathetic and took less than five minutes to put my makeup on. Because I'd been forced to read hundreds of books for my job, I knew enough about a wide range of subjects to be a sparkling conversationalist when I wanted to be. I had funny, interesting friends. I had one of the coolest jobs in Portland. I'd taken a fellatio class.

I brought a lot to the table. But I also brought my ass to the table, and in my mind, it was so huge that it shattered the table into tiny shards and then nobody had anything on the table because there was no table.

Weight is a powerful thing.

I remember watching *The Truth About Cats and Dogs* back in the '90s and seeing size 10 Janeane Garofolo playing "the fat one" and thinking, *I will never be thin enough to be the fat girl in a movie.*[2]

And I will never be thin enough to be attractive to men.

Ruminating on dangerously, pathologically wrongheaded thoughts like these led me to be a thirty-four-year-old virgin and to avoid relationships for a decade after my first breakup.

I knew that something was broken. Something is still broken.

I've always known it, but I hadn't had the courage or temerity to do anything about it until my OFW year. More precisely, until I started dating Scott and realized that no matter how great my romantic life got, as long as I felt like my ass crushed all my other awesome table offerings, I would forever believe that someone who wasn't as fat as me was doing me a favor by dating me. It was time to do something.

I'd been so impressed with how Samantha Hess (the professional cuddler) had educated herself out of her body issues that I decided to research ways to do the same. I went to search for *healing your relationship with your body* and Google autocompleted my sentence to *healing*

---

2   If you haven't seen it, it's another modernized Cyrano story, but this was Hollywood and Cyrano was a woman, so instead of a giant nose, she was cursed with a hideously medium-size body.

your relationship with your mother. I bookmarked some of those results and moved on.

Here's a frustrating thing I've run into over and over again: There are clinics and groups for anorexics and bulimics and there are hospitals that offer surgery to those who are beyond morbidly obese, but for those of us who are "just" compulsive overeaters and obese, there really aren't any programs, or if there are, those programs aren't paid for by insurance unless it gets to the point where you need a gastric bypass. It's like going to a doctor with stage two colon cancer and having her say, "We're sorry, but we can't offer you any treatment until you get to stage four."[3]

After a lot of searching, I finally found a combination class / therapy group taught by a woman named Jacci Jones, whose name sounds like a badass lady cop with something to prove, but she's actually a soft-spoken, sweet marriage and family therapist with something to prove...about disordered eating. The group focused on food addiction and healing one's relationship with food, and of course my insurance didn't pay for it, but thankfully I was making enough freelancing to afford to pay out of pocket. Insurance companies need to stop being stupid about weight. And mental illness. And pretty much everything else.

---

3   To be clear, being overweight does *not* automatically mean you're not healthy. Those people who shame fat people because they claim to be concerned about their health need to realize that it's absolutely possible to retain your health as an obese person with exercise, the right foods, or just good genes. But for me, because I ate terrible foods and didn't exercise, obesity meant gallstones, high blood pressure, pre-diabetes, a bad back, and the beginnings of fatty liver disease. Obesity and health didn't go together for me.

I told myself that I was going to either lose weight in the group or come to a place of peace with whatever my body looked like and not continue to torture myself by trying to get smaller instead of healthier.

My only concern about the group was the term *food addiction*. I'd never thought of myself as an addict, but once I started going to the group, I realized that of course I was.

I remember at one point talking about how much power a Reese's Peanut Butter Cup had over me and later thinking about how insane that sentence had been. I thought about the peanut butter cup on the counter in its orange plastic wrapper. It was just sitting there, being inanimate. Did I believe peanut butter cups had brains? Souls? Diabolical plans to get inside my belly?

The first thing I learned in group was that no food is inherently good or bad. It just is what it is and it has whatever caloric and nutritional content it has. And what you choose to do with food, on its own or in combination with other foods, can have an immediate positive or negative effect on your health and mood.

Pretty simple stuff, but once you truly connect to that idea, it's quite powerful.

The group also helped me learn to fight with my brain more effectively. For the majority of my adult life, I'd spent my free time thinking about all the things I'd done wrong so far and all the things that would go wrong in the future. What I was learning now was that thinking something didn't make it true. Another very simple idea, but for someone for whom being right was a constant imperative, this was a profound and liberating thought.

It feels counterintuitive, but in order to begin to heal from a lifetime of envisioning worst-case scenarios, I had to learn not to trust myself sometimes. Because an anxious brain is the ultimate unreliable narrator.

In the past, when I'd been under stress or feeling regret for a binge, my inner voice came at me with laser efficiency.

Look what you did to yourself. You're disgusting.

Why are you so weak? You're like a child.

You're gonna die alone, and that's what you deserve.

This is why I filled my time alone with a constant stream of social media, sudoku, naps, or videos of cats falling off things. Because no one wants to hang out with that asshole.

The group taught me to do the opposite of what one would normally do to a person with that voice—it taught me to empathize with it. To ask what had turned her into such a raging bitch. To ask what she might be afraid of.

Turns out, she's afraid I'm going to have a massive heart attack. She's afraid I'm going to be uncomfortably heavy and miserable for the rest of my life. She's afraid I'll die alone.

She—that voice—is like the shitty, cruel, misguided mother I never had.[4] She believes that even though the insults have never worked— not one single time—she needs to continue haranguing me every day

---

4   As I was growing up, my mother was a casserole-making, terrible-school-play-attending, Christmas-elf-impersonating hundred-pound ball of energy and acceptance. She came from a long line of weight-obsessed women but never said anything to me about mine. Partially because our family was very adept at avoiding uncomfortable conversations. Remember that game "the ground is poison," where you leap around on pillows and laundry and furniture to avoid touching the floor? We played "conflict is poison" during my entire childhood.

so that I won't make the same mistakes over and over again. Sure, she's wildly ineffective, but she's scrappy.

The voice didn't totally stop once I understood where she was coming from, but I was periodically able to reason with her.

> VOICE: Look at your thighs. You make me sick.
> ME: Hey, Dick. [I call her Dick.] Listen, I understand why you're concerned about them, but they're doing their job really well. See how they're holding me up and stuff?
> DICK: They're so jiggly and gross.
> ME: Well, your exoskeleton is made of bile and cat poop, and live bees fly out of your mouth every time you speak, but you seem to get around okay.
> DICK: That's a low blow.
> ME: I'm just saying we have stuff in common.

Over just a few months, the group had slipped me little pieces of information that, along with my sitting in a room for two hours and talking about food issues once a week, began to gain a foothold in my previously embattled brain.

We had a nutritionist come in who told us that sugar was linked to brain fog, and I went off sugary treats for the first time in my adult life, which balanced out my moods, and while it didn't lift the fog, it definitely thinned it out a little.

We watched a video from a doctor who informed us that walking for thirty minutes a day reduced the risk of heart attack by 31 percent—31 percent!

This information, which I imagine had been out there in the world for quite a while but which I'd been ignoring because Reese's Peanut Butter Cups were actively sabotaging me, felt revolutionary. In order to become healthy, I'd always pictured myself in one of those "getting strong now" film montages, where I started off chubby and had someone yelling at me in the rain to do pull-ups and sit-ups and bench-press a large log and pull a tractor tire with a huge chain while I cried nonstop and screamed, "I've got nowhere else to go!" But this idea that I could stroll my way to health? That I could meander my way out of a heart attack? That made health appear attainable. Because I have a low threshold for misery.

Two months later, my brother and I started a bet with two other friends that involved us going to the gym three days a week. I had to post real-time pictures of myself entering the gym and then leaving it at least twenty-five minutes later. I would owe the other three participants thirty-three dollars each for every week I failed.

We were all so clearly annoyed in the photos of the first few weeks that my roommate Shelly, who was in on the bet, texted, *If someone came upon these texts and didn't read English, they'd think we were a group of friends who had bonded over a shared hatred of mall architecture.*

The bet was a success. I started walking three days a week without fail and have done so for a year now.

We're still engaged in the bet and I'm still working on trying to be healthy rather than thin. It's a struggle, but for the first time, I have hope that I won't wake up every day for the rest of my life thinking about how I fucked up with food yesterday and wondering how I'm going to fuck up with it today. Food doesn't feel like my enemy or my savior anymore, and if I gain a few pounds, it's not the worst tragedy in the history of the universe. It's just a thing that happens.

I've forgiven myself for all my food-related sins, but even more than that, I've realized that there's no such thing as a food-related sin; there's just eating that will make me feel good and eating that will make me feel bad. And neither choice has a damned thing to do with my character.

I'm flawed, but I'm trying, and I can finally see the beauty and humanity in both of those things.

Where work is concerned, I still haven't decided what I want to do when I grow up. I'm currently teaching writing and storytelling to adults and high-school kids, writing columns for which I don't do a damn thing that scares me, and doing some freelance advertising work. Now that I'm out of the weekly dread-terror-relief cycle that *Live Wire!* used to cause, I'm not in a huge hurry to figure it all out.

I still perform, but now I know very clearly which experiences will bring me joy (reading essays, telling stories) and which will not (situations in which I am paired with a genius and must ask questions that may expose me as a nongenius).

I've defined for myself which relationships I should spend time thinking about (the kind with the people I love) and which I shouldn't (the kind with four hundred strangers).

I also discovered that I should seek work in a field in which neuroticism is a plus (I would make a great Chihuahua, for instance).

When I look back on my year of living (relatively) dangerously, I'm half shocked that it was me who did those things and half shocked that I'd been so scared to do them.

Things I did that I'll never do again: get a Brazilian, allow a stranger to put her vagina on my freshly washed clothing, have public

299

sex, get stoned, and rate human beings like they're shitty brunch spots on Yelp.

Things I did that I hope I'll never do again: pee on the floor of someone I'm trying to impress.

Things I did that I might do again: leave a job when it causes a constant stream of cortisol to flow through my veins, go to a cuddler (if my boyfriend weirdly stops touching me), and attend a water aerobics class when I need encouragement from the elderly.

As for how my year-and-a-half-long adventure affected me, it didn't magically change my entire life. I'm not a whole new me. I'm not fearless.

But I did learn that when it comes to increasing one's general level of pluck, you don't have to bungee-jump off a bridge—or even jump off the high dive, for that matter.

It turns out, grand gestures aren't necessary. Because every time you dip your toe outside your comfort zone, you nudge its border just a little. And a little is enough to change things a lot.

My life isn't enormously different, but in addition to finally being okay with leaving *Live Wire!*, I found that one small, important thing did change for me. Just one word.

Interesting.

When someone suggests I try something new, something that sounds like it could lead to awkwardness or discomfort or risk, instead of *That sounds terrifying,* my brain now says, *Well. That sounds interesting.*

It doesn't say, *Let's fucking do it! We are totally gonna turn this* [mildly adventurous experience] *into our bitch!* But it does offer up a surprisingly judgment-neutral response, which is kind of a big deal.

I wanted to make myself more optimistic, and I feel like my one shiny new word absolutely counts. It's tiny, but it counts. And I spent a whole year doing weird shit without having made that infinitesimal shift, so it turns out you don't have to be optimistic to live an interesting life.

So if I came away from this whole thing with a lesson, I guess it's this: Fuck optimism. I mean, I love optimism, and if you have it naturally, that's wonderful. Go with that, always and forever. You're lucky and I hate you a little.

If you don't have it naturally yet you go ahead and do the thing that's going to make your life—and, by extension, *you*—more interesting, well, you're still doing it, aren't you? You're still doing it with your Okay Fine Whatever attitude, which is a lot more of an accomplishment, if you ask me.

So go forth, and do things hesitantly! Say, *Hey, world! I don't trust that you have my best interests at heart, but I'm willing to do this anyway! I just want to be clear that I'm not promising to like it! World? Are you still listening?*

The thing is, the world probably isn't listening. The world is just minding its own business, spinning at a thousand miles an hour and trying to hold it together, just like you are.

So this is going to be on you.

Do it.

Roll your eyes, throw a mini-tantrum, say it's gonna suck balls, and do it.

And just know, somewhere, I'm saying it's gonna suck balls and doing it too.

Acknowledgments

(Or: Sorry I Didn't See You for Two Years; I Hope We Can Have a Drink Now and Catch Up. You Look Great!)

It is a goddamned miracle that you're holding this book. Writing it was the strangest blend of joy and hideous torture and it would not exist without an army of supportive, forgiving, generous people who believed that I was capable of doing it even when I told them they were full of shit, which I'd like to apologize for here. And also thank them.

Thanks, first, to my agent Laurie Fox for seeing that my column was a book and for pestering me (charmingly) until I let go of the fear and wrote the fucking thing. To Reagan Arthur and the amazing team at Little, Brown and to Jean Garnett for having faith in my work, the keenest of editing eyes, and the patience not to kill me or the project. To Greg Kulick for a beautiful cover and Tracy Roe for slogging through the grammatical nightmare that was this book. To Laura Velasquez, Maggie Southard, and the entire marketing and publicity

303

team. And to Christine McKinley, without whom this book wouldn't exist. Thank you for nudging me.

To Allison Picard for building me up (along with every other person in her life).

To Shelly Caldwell for being unendingly generous and patient and the best housemate in the history of the world.

To the girls, Marie Murphy, Shelley McLendon, and Erin O'Regan, for always supporting me and still being my friends even when I disappeared for months at a time and then showed up only to whine and eat a lot of your cheese.

Tips on escaping a car trunk are courtesy of Chelsea Cain, who is always there with helpful advice and a bottle of something.

To members of my various writers' groups: Cynthia Whitcomb, Marc Acito, Daniel Wilson, Scott Poole, Stacy Bolt, Ryan White, Rachel Bachmann, and Storm Large.

To Tobey and Teri Fitch, who offered me their house on Vashon, their faith, and an ongoing series of perfectly cooked meats.

To Fiona McCann (who gave me the gift of a reason to write every week), Byron Beck, Zach Dundas, and Cornelius Swart.

To some extraordinary writer friends who helped me imagine this was possible: Cheryl Strayed, Karen Karbo, Mike Sacks, Kathleen Lane, and Lidia Yuknavitch.

To Jason Rouse, Sean McGrath, and Andrew Harris for being effortlessly funny every day.

To Robyn Tenenbaum, Jim Brunberg, and Kate Sokoloff at *Live Wire!* for their patience and faith in me.

To Luke Burbank and Ophira Eisenberg for being so forthcoming, and to Todd Schultz for being so smart.

ACKNOWLEDGMENTS

To my readers Jamie and Phil Incorvia, Dr. Jessica Duffett, Courtenay Rudzinski, Kari Fiori, and Julie Livingston, whom I would highly recommend as a book editor if that was what she wanted to be, which she doesn't, so don't even ask.

To Stephan Cassell for his marketing brains and Nick Wichman and Karen Wippich for their generosity and talent.

To every man I dated during that insane year: You were so sweet. Most of you. Except that one guy. What was up with him?

To Jake Shivery for being essentially responsible for my career as an essayist. Sorry about that.

To Jennifer Blinder and the whole Byrd family and the circus tent of extraordinary people who come with them.

To my whole extended family, but especially Bob and Sandi Hameister and Cheri and John Michael, who have always supported my creative endeavors.

And to Scott Charters for loving me, for fixing my driver's-side mirror, for not making more incontinence jokes than you did, for doing sex with me a lot, and for being such a good character in my book. I love you. And it's not just because you're tall. But that's part of it.

About the Author

Courtenay Hameister is a professional nervous person. During her twelve years as host and head writer for *Live Wire!*, a nationally syndicated public radio show, she interviewed more than five hundred intimidating people and wrote two hundred personal essays in bursts of anxiety-fueled inspiration the night before each show. Her work has also been featured in *McSweeney's*, APM's *Marketplace*, *More*, and some scathing e-mails to the customer-service department at Macy's.